Apply the Secret to Lose Weight

Rafik Romdhane

ISBN: 9798388405982

Dedication

To my two sons, Zakary Romdhane and William Romdhane. I love you guys a lot.

Acknowledgment

Our bodies are holy vessels that house our souls so we may live on the earthly plane. The body requires nourishment, respect, healing, and activities that promote its optimal functioning.

About the Author

Through a comprehensive breakthrough and long-term weight loss method, Rafik Romdhane rewires the subconscious to focus on what truly matters, breaking the mold for weight loss. He shows how to reshape one's mind by paying attention to thoughts in his book, which changes how you live and eat. This can lead to a happier, healthier life.

Since the diet culture has merged into a system of beliefs that are ingrained in society, he'd like to help a lot of people feel better about themselves. He wants to help them lose weight and look amazing by freeing themselves.

The book has psychology tips for maintaining a constant sense of self, nutrition advice, stress management tips, and motivation for managing your nutrition. Using his own experience, Rafik gives readers advice on how to reclaim their bodies, minds, and lives.

To avoid a bad relationship with food, he encourages readers to rethink how they feel about themselves, their bodies, and food, unlike diet culture. In his story, he tells how he lost weight successfully by overcoming negative belief patterns.

The English version of his book will be released in January 2023, and translations will follow.

Growing up in Tunisia, Rafik liked playing football a lot. While Rafik loves the Mediterranean Sea and spending time at the beach, he decided 25 years ago to move to Montreal, Canada, for the biggest adventure of his life, along with his two sons.

Contents

Preface

Chapter 1: Alignment

Changing how your mind works can transform your life.

It can profoundly change the way you think, feel and behave. Thinking deeply enriches your life and encourages deeper living.

To think deeply means to think beyond your limitation of beliefs, preconceived ideas, and prevailing opinions. It means to shed off false convictions so that the truth can unfold.

The problem is that we haven't really learned how to think in a way that benefits us. Our thoughts are unfocused, mostly superficial, and not directed.

Our thoughts simply come to us randomly, without conscious effort. At the same time, we don't use our thinking processes to think deeply voluntarily.

We no longer seek to think beyond our own set boundaries and comfort zones.

Most of us are perfectly happy within the comfortable confines of our own beliefs, attitudes, and prejudices. We remain stuck within the mire of our own thought loops. We rarely think about breaking out and broadening our horizons.

There's a little secret that you should know. You may have heard the secret to living a happy life with purpose and productivity.

Do you want to have a more positive life? Maybe you want to be more successful in your career or have a fulfilling relationship.

All great philosophers, high achievers, and present thinkers agree on this simple truth.

"Thought is the fount of action, life, and manifestation; make the fountain pure, and all will be pure."

Life consists mainly of the storm of thoughts that is forever flowing through one's head. Brilliant minds have tried discovering the secret to living a happy and purposeful life. You, too, should try to find it.

You may be a bit skeptical at first, which is understandable. There have been a few people who are manipulators of this concept that have misled people for the sake of the monetary game.

You can be the judge for yourself. You know, we all live in a world full of thought. And our thoughts create our experiences and perspectives. Meaning we experience what we think. The majority of our thoughts throughout the day don't influence our behavior or cause harm or repeated thoughts.

The ones we think about repeatedly can begin to shape our reality and affect our actions, behavior, and our attitudes. If we have quality positive thoughts, we create the quality in our life that is positive.

Now, are you unhappy with your life?

Most unhappy people seek to change things in their life. We believe that changing or transforming our environment will bring the revolution we want and hope to see.

Unhappy people seek out substances to desensitize or numb the mind. But this only is temporary. Some seek to travel to escape their problems, and others will buy material things for momentary happiness.

The cycle repeats if you continue to change your environment to be happy. We assume that change starts from the outside. We usually forget that the environment does play a small role in changing your situation.

The environment makes you feel the way you do. It would be best if you first changed your thought process. Only then will the outside change.

Your thinking directly correlates to how you feel and how your body reacts.

Negative thinking can cause anxiety and depression symptoms. Your thoughts influence how you feel and how you feel impacts how you act. You are what you think.

Eckhart Tolle said.

"If you get the inside right, the outside will fall into place."

Repeated thoughts reinforce what you believe. The more you do something, the more likely you will do it again in the future.

Repetition rewires the brain and breeds habits. The more the neurons fire together, the more likely they will fire together in the future.

And neurosciences say cells that fire together wire together, meaning the more we repeat the same thought over and over in our head, it slowly creates a new neuronal path. It slowly becomes a habit that is hard to break.

When we think of a thought, our brain creates a chemical reaction and then triggers any motion. A new circuit is made within our brain, and it sends a signal to our body, and we react a certain way.

There are several ways you can change your mindset. The topmost task you should consider doing is determining your mindset. When you have a goal, you want to achieve it. Ask yourself and push your limits.

"What mindset do I need, as well as people who were successful at this goal? What was their mindset?"

Change yourself and avoid detrimental self-talk. When you tell yourself that you're not good enough, your thoughts will reshape your reality to match these counteractive thoughts, and you'll be held back from the life you want.

Start by changing your negative self-talk to 'I am good enough' or 'I can do this,' and don't forget, 'I love myself.' It may sound weird, but it will really help you transform your life!

You should also try to surround yourself with like-minded people. When you are around negative people, their negativity will run off on you.

Find positive, uplifting people and learn how to think and modify their habits and mindset to yours. This also means that you should consider setting protective boundaries with the individuals that are not acting for your highest good.

Next, you must learn to get out of your comfort zone. Challenge yourself to do new things which will cause you to rise to the occasion and change your mindset.

Question your thinking and positively reframe your negative thoughts. Doing this will help reduce stress, and you will develop a feeling of motivation.

The quality of our thoughts creates the quality of our life; our thoughts create experiences, and we experience what we think. Remind yourself often that the power of your thoughts will become your beliefs. Thoughts have power.

We already know that the way we think has a huge impact on our life outcomes, but is it possible to affect our food choices as well?

The short answer to that is YES!!!

Our thoughts can influence our food choices, whether they're positive or negative.

People start to notice that something's wrong when they feel uncomfortable or in a bad mood. That's why they concentrate on what's close to them right now.

This kind of thinking makes us pay attention to the sensory qualities of food instead of what's abstract, like how nourishing it is.

The same goes for a good mood. When people are happy, they can focus on the more abstract aspects of food, like how healthy it is.

Every time you hear yourself saying something negative about yourself, stop and force yourself to say something positive because negativity is real, and it happens every single day.

We are what we think about and what we intend. Our thoughts and intentions manifest into reality. Have you noticed that food prepared with love and positive thoughts tastes very good?

There is nothing like eating good food to make your day better. People usually change their minds once they try something. Sometimes, they even learn to love something.

Our brains are constantly going through feelings of love and wanting things. There's a specific vibration going on that keeps you stuck.

A vibrational variance happens when you want something and believe in it. When you want something and believe in something else, then there's again a vibrational variance that drives the metabolism.

You can accept that everything is vibrational, at least conceptually. Keep in mind that everything you see is a vibrational interpretation.

A vibrational interpretation is what you perceive with your 5 senses: what you hear with your ears, a vibrational interpretation of what your fingertips do, a vibrational interpretation of what your nose does, and a vibrational interpretation of what you taste and smell.

You're all vibrational. All your cells are made of vibrations. Even the food that we eat is vibrational. Our very core, our essence, and our existence are based on atoms - and the core function of atoms is to vibrate.

Getting angry at someone is a vibrational disagreement. You understand that it doesn't resonate with you.

When you feel something, you know you're in alignment. You're not perfect. Nobody is. It's okay to say what you feel.

A lot of people express themselves through their diets. If you feel guilty eating something, what does that tell you about your relationship with yourself?

There's nothing wrong with it in and of itself. You're going to find food delectable in a way that you've never known it to be.

Lots of people eat a lot of food to try to compensate for the disconnect between who they are and who they let themselves be.

You can make food more satisfying by blending food properties with similar vibrations because combining foods with similar vibrations will provide you with a much better meal.

A food's vibration affects not just its taste but also extends to how it feels to you, how it tastes, and what it does for your body. But there's a lot more that affects food's vibration.

Vibration can only be fully understood by preparing your own frequency in your own physical body and asking what you're participating in to join that frequency. Food is one of the most cooperative things in that process.

When we associate food with 'bad,' we're not fully allowing the natural digestive process to take place. The mind-gut connection is strong. Therefore, when we associate food with 'bad,' we're limiting the body's ability to digest.

Stomach acid that is generally produced in high amounts when we smell and chew our food won't be produced in as high amounts, resulting in the slowing of the emptying of the stomach.

From here, we find there is an increased risk of bloating and changed bowel motions. The more that we can stimulate proper stomach acid and kickstart the whole digestive process, the fewer digestive symptoms will be experienced.

The cycle we experience with negative self-talk and emotional eating directly results from the way our brain remembers the actions that made us feel really awesome and good.

So, when we experience thoughts and situations that make us feel bad or down, our brain tells us to seek what made us feel good before, driving us to eat and indulge again. If you repeat this process enough times, it will eventually become automatic.

Chapter 2: Shift your vibration

You are a living energy field. Your body is composed of energy-producing particles, each of which is in constant motion. So, like everything and everyone else in the universe, you are vibrating and creating energy.

The field of vibrational medicine, sometimes called energy medicine, seeks to use the vibrational energy generated by and around your body to optimize your health. To many people, the concept of energy fields in the body may sound more spiritual than medicinal.

More research must be done to understand how electrical and magnetic energy in the body stimulate chemical processes. But there's growing evidence that these energies can be used to influence your health outcomes.

But what is vibrational energy? Have you ever tried thinking about it?

Vibrations are a kind of rhythm. Rhythms happen on a grand scale, like seasonal changes and tidal patterns. They also happen within your body.

Heartbeats, breathing rates, and circadian rhythms are examples of physiological rhythms we can see, feel, and measure.

But there are much smaller vibrations happening in your body, too. Inside each one of your cells, molecules vibrate at characteristic rates.

These vibrations generate electromagnetic energy waves. Researchers have found that vibrations and the electromagnetic energy associated with them cause changes in your cells, which can then affect how your body functions.

Have you ever felt like your mind and the reality around you are in sync? After paying close attention, you may notice that shifting my thinking will change the outcome of my life.

It's no accident that positive and grateful people attract more positive situations to be grateful for. More and more people are starting to realize the direct impact that their mind activity has on their reality.

Our minds emit vibrations that are constantly at work. Just like thunder and lightning, radio waves, and ultraviolet rays, a thought vibrates through the mind and manifests into reality whether we're aware of it or not.

People get good at mastering their thoughts, and most people can learn to control how they think. Manifesting happiness, joy, health, wealth, freedom, and happiness in a tangible way is possible with the right mindset frequency.

Nikola Tesla once said, *"If you wish to understand the universe, think in terms of energy, frequency, and vibration."*

There is vibration in everything. The earth, the sky, the wind, fire, and water all vibrate. Our physical body, our organs, blood, all animals, trees, flowers, rivers, the ocean, stones, crystals, and metal all vibrate.

Any matter in our universe, whether visible or unseen, can be broken down and analyzed into its purest, most basic form.

It's basically pure energy or light that resonates and exists as a vibratory frequency. The building blocks of everything in our world are all the same, and when science breaks down matter into its smallest parts, energy vibrates at different frequencies. It's a fact.

Some people call this The Law of Attraction or The Law of Vibration; it really doesn't matter what you call it as long as you are aware of it and respect it as a universal law, just like we understand and respect the law of gravity.

People are usually confused about how vibrational energy can impact our lives. Well, a simple answer to that is man, as a mechanical system, is extremely complex and his mechanical properties readily undergo change.

The effect of vibration on the human body as a mechanical and biological system is a very complex phenomenon. There is limited reliable information on the magnitude of the forces required to produce mechanical damage to the human body.

As humans, we are exposed to constant energy. What sets everything apart in our internal and external world are two things: the atomic structure and the vibrational frequency of what we focus on.

The speed or frequency of these vibrations determines whether something appears as a solid, liquid, or gas.

The frequency levels of frequencies that we are exposed to trigger a response in our bodies, and the signals that our bodies transmit to our brains are triggered by all the energies we have been exposed to.

Whenever we talk about a person, situation, or setting's "vibe," we mean a vibration, which we then categorize as positive or negative.

The way people feel, how they see the world, and how they feel about themselves are all things that influence their energy. Our belief systems and sense of self are shaped by how we've dealt with life experiences.

A positive vibration is a high-frequency thinking pattern, attitude, and feeling, whereas a negative vibration is a low-frequency thinking pattern, attitude, or feeling.

It's easy to identify a negative vibration if you know when and how you feel resistance. Positive vibrations make us feel at ease, whereas negative vibrations can make us feel doubtful, worried, and anxious.

We also pick up energies that don't belong to us. When we begin to identify these energies as part of who we are, we get stuck in a low vibrational state. It's time we let go of this resistance and live according to our inner peace.

The following image is of a model:

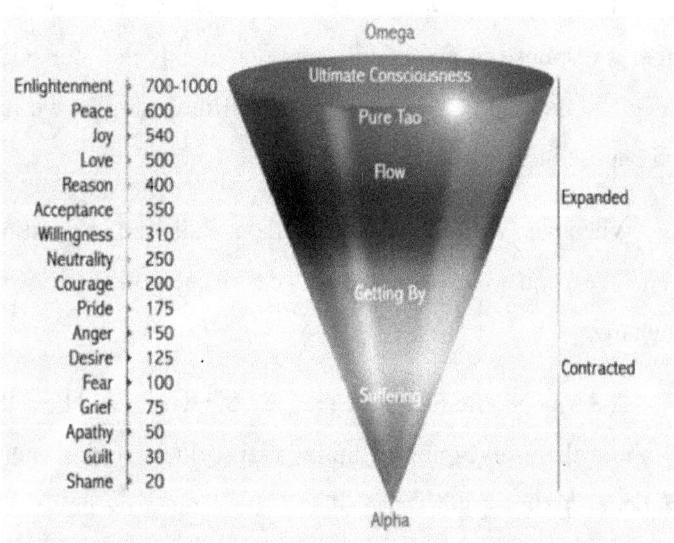

The model developed in the 70s by the psychiatrist Dr. David Hawkins has a scale of states of energy (called Levels of consciousness) from 20 to 1000, which can help us to evaluate our daily vibrational state.

It's a good tool to get unstuck and raise our vibrations.

Shifting the tone of your internal dialogue is key. Your body and mind react to the vibrations of your thoughts.

When you talk to yourself in a positive tone, you will immediately experience an immediate shift in vibration. Pay attention to what you are saying to yourself because, at the end of the day, you are the one creating your own reality.

We live in a world of thought. Our thoughts create our experiences; thus, we experience what we think. It is the quality of our thoughts, then, that creates the quality of our life. When we're unhappy where we are in life, we seek to create change.

So we go about transforming our environment, believing that doing so will create the necessary change we hope to see.

We buy things for a materialistic boost of happiness. We travel to escape our problems. We seek substances to numb the mind and help us forget.

But of course, we fall back to where we had started: unhappy with where we are today. And so the cycle repeats itself.

We buy, we travel, we forget—always focusing on the external factors we need to alter in order to create better circumstances.

Thoughts, in and of themselves, have no power—it's only when we actively invest our attention into them that they begin to seem real.

And when we engage with specific thoughts, we begin to feel the emotions that were triggered by these thoughts—we enter a new emotional state which then influences how we act.

Thoughts trigger emotions, and the vibrational frequency of these emotions then feeds back into the original thought.

And as we continue to give mental attention to the initial thought, it reaffirms the emotion, which then energizes the thought. And so we experience a continuous cycle of think, feel, think, feel, think, feel.

This is how your thoughts create your reality. It's in the way you behave and act that you define who you are and what you experience in life and the way you behave and act is simply a construction of how you think, feel, and do. This includes changing your thoughts about food.

Everything you do requires that you make a choice. When to get up, what to wear, and what to watch on television are all daily decisions that shape us. Often, we fall into habits because we prefer certain options.

Maybe you watch Game of Thrones every night because it always entertains you, or perhaps you wear sparkly green eyeshadow because it makes you feel glamorous. While it can feel secure to have some reliable, tried-and-true options, it is unrealistic to make them your only ones.

Not every preference fits every situation, and it would be inappropriate to not change your decisions when you're in a different environment or circumstance. Food exists by the same rules.

Of course, it's natural to have a favorite dessert or restaurant. But if specific foods become your only options, your mindset might be one of obsession.

Rigid habits, such as only eating certain foods, can quickly turn your preferences into positions and leave you stuck.

You should enjoy the foods you consume but not worship them. You should not be afraid of what you are eating.

Flexibility, exhibited through the willingness to forego a preference temporarily, is an essential aspect of a healthy relationship with food.

Foods can make you feel afraid, anxious, or uncomfortable eating. The fear of food may come from irrational thoughts about how it impacts your body or weight or from negative memories of food.

The frequency of a healthy human body is usually anywhere between 62-78 Hz. The food that we eat, the thoughts we think, the environment in which we live, and many other factors have an impact on our vibrational frequency.

We have all experienced going to a certain place where something didn't feel quite right. After some time, we started feeling depleted and drained.

No one can claim to feel energized and refreshed after a night of processed food and alcoholic drinks. Or after you have had a heated debate with someone.

This is because the exchange of energy is constantly happening. All items, places, and people that are vibrating at a lower frequency impact our own frequency in a negative way.

The absence of strict rules surrounding eating and food habits is another key aspect of having a healthy relationship with food. Instead of seeing deviations from preferred foods as a judgment of oneself or their worth, there is more of a tendency to go with the flow and accept deviations as a natural part of life.

Some foods are deemed "good" and "clean," while others are deemed "bad" or "junk." These labels make us feel in control. In reality, they don't mean much at all.

They're constructs that make people feel bad about their food choices and proud of theirs. On most days, you're going to eat both "healthy" and "unhealthy" things, and that's fine.

One thing you should remember is that there are some foods that have different vibrations than others. There is a big difference between the strength and the vibration of vegetables.

You understand the energy-giving value of food. When you are in a vulnerable or angry vibration, you match up with things that are not well-being in nature and vice versa.

This is the starting place where we want to talk about receptive mode elation, appreciation, love, vulnerability, insecurity, and anger.

You've been chasing the energy of your vortex for so long, and that's how you have to align yourself. This is what is known as the force of creation, and it's the driving force of your creation.

So if you align yourself with it, it creates a better you. You can move more powerfully when you align yourself with this frequency because it's the energy that's coming from all your desires and sensations.

This is the fastest way to move because there's no second, it's infinite, and it's never-ending.

Chapter 3: The Secret

Is there something that is capable of dividing and connecting people from all walks of life with the same degree of strength?

Our beliefs.

We're one conviction away from a global awakening. If everybody shared one belief on a universal scope of respect for fellow humans without needing anything from them, we'd change everything.

How can something that has no substance, no pulse, no blood, or life control whether or not we live in harmony with each other if it doesn't have a pulse, blood, or life?

I hope to clarify the essence of this often revered and highly controversial topic in this chapter, which can border on being an addiction or being a common day prejudicial practice depending on who's talking about it.

A belief is neither safe nor deadly. The truth is that beliefs are merely a manifestation of one's environment.

Beliefs are metaphorical manifestations of where we have lived, the people who were there, and what they said, thought, and did.

As mankind has evolved, it has always become better.

Some brave souls stood up to traditional values and traditional discriminatory principles, providing reasonable doubts about them, even if they weren't on a global level.

My perspective on this topic hasn't always been the same as it is today. In any case, I imagine I am not alone. I connect daily with people from all over the world through different social media platforms.

People should keep fighting for change. It doesn't always happen instantly. It usually happens over time. Those who are open to it are usually fighting for it to happen, and they've evolved along the way.

Evolution doesn't work in the way that some people think it does, so they adapt to it after it happens. People don't have to give up core values and principles just because they stand up for different beliefs and ideas. To me, it means they've embraced the ones they've reached out to from their own convictions.

There's nothing sweet and sweet about the mind. In addition to what I just mentioned, it also brought about superstition, slavery, and war. So, that makes it more puzzling the way human thought works.

It's the same mind, with the same powers of thought, that created science, philosophy, and art millennium after millennium, mired in archaic social formations, bound by irrational superstitions.

Think about something simple, like the belief that there is coke in the fridge. But that's just one kind of thought. And suppose you want one. That's also a thought. It's basically a desire.

A belief is a statement about how things work or how they don't work. It's the kind of thing that can be true or false. Hopefully, we believe things more than we don't. If they don't, it's rational to change them to fit with the world.

Alternatively, desires don't represent the world. For instance, we don't say that my desire for coke is false just because I don't have one. But we do say that my desire is unsatisfied when you don't have one. You must change the world if you are going to fulfill a desire.

Intentions are the third type of thought we need to fulfill our desires. You might come up with a new kind of thought if you believe there is a coke in the fridge and you really want a coke.

That thought is known as an intention. An intention can make you get off your duff, make you walk over to the refrigerator, and pick up your coke. Or it might not if you are weak-willed or lazy.

In order to understand the power of thought and its impact on the world, we need first to understand its power.

By understanding how beliefs represent or misrepresent the way the world is, how desires set forth possible changes to the world, and how intentions motivate us to change the world, we will have a better understanding of how we might change it.

There may seem to be a lot to do with that, but it is actually much simpler than it appears at first since beliefs, desires, and intentions are all constructed of the same basic building blocks -- just put together differently. A concept or an idea is the basis for all of them.

For example, my belief that there is coke in the fridge, my desire to drink a coke, and my intention to get a coke all involve the concept or idea of coke.

We can begin to understand the power of thought by examining the nature of concepts and ideas, where they come from, and how they can be combined to create such a wide variety of thoughts if we consider them in this way. Once we understand this, we can begin to explore what different types of thoughts do.

A great number of the most accomplished people of our time were viewed by experts as having no future by them, such as Charles Darwin, Lucille Ball, Marcel Proust, and many others.

Yet, like all great achievers from Mozart to Einstein, they developed their abilities over time. I would like to leave you with this key insight: when we realize that we can change our own abilities when we have a growth mindset, we can take our game to another level.

In what ways does a growth mindset accomplish this?

In fact, it has been shown that mindset has physiological manifestations. Brain scans reveal that people with fixed mindsets are more active when they receive feedback about their performance, such as grades.

On the other hand, those with a growth mindset become most active when they receive information about improving their performance.

An individual with a fixed mindset is most concerned about their judgment, while an individual with a growth mindset is more concerned with their learning.

Also, the mindset has other consequences: people with a fixed mindset see effort as a bad thing, something only the weakest need, while those with a growth mindset see effort as what makes us smart, as what makes us smart. When people with a fixed mindset face setbacks or failures, they tend to think they're incapable.

So they lose interest or withdraw. That's what we see as motivational fatigue. Behind it is a fixed mindset, whereas people with a growth mindset understand that setbacks are part of growth, so they find ways around them.

Do you know that there is a philosophy that suggests you can manifest your deepest desires into being with merely the power of thought?

We know it by the name 'the Law of Attraction, and it is one of the cosmic forces that are working around us without us knowing about them.

"What you see in your reality now are the seeds, i.e., the thoughts and emotions, you planted at a certain point in your life."

-Maria Concha.

Your current life - from your home and partner to your career - is all a consequence of your thoughts. Pay attention, and you'll see how your thoughts reflect what you're experiencing. This is manifestation.

Your experiences are attracted to you since the Law of Attraction responds to your thoughts at some point. When you focus on a particular person or thing, you create a vibrational pull that attracts them to you.

Being conscious of my thoughts instead of reacting to them means being aware of them.

When you focus on something in the present moment, whether it's remembering a past event, observing something in the present, or imagining a future event, the Law of Attraction responds to it.

Your desire will attract what you focus on into your life, according to the Law of Attraction. Whatever you can imagine is possible if you put forth a plan for getting there.

It's a great law of attraction that says that like attracts like. If you give your energy and attention to something, it's going to come back to you.

In this abundant universe, the Law of Attraction governs everything. You're being guided by universal forces right now to finally understand how to manifest everything that you put your mind to. It doesn't discriminate. It only exists with perfection.

It's true that every moment of your life is creating your own reality. With every conscious act, you create your present and your future. Any goal you set in your mind is achievable, but only if you put it into practice.

Your thoughts will attract bad outcomes if you focus on them. When you think positively, have goals, and have a plan, you will manifest them.

You'll gravitate to things, people, or situations that have the same energy as you do too. It'll only amp up your vibration, whether you're positive or negative.

Depending on what you read, you can get different interpretations of the law of attraction, but it has a few foundational behaviors. The first one is a mindset, and the other is action. Some theories claim that focusing intently creates a pull between you and what you want.

We make that happen through growth and action, not just wishful thinking. You have to bring your whole self to everything you do, professionally and personally.

Our mental fitness demands setting goals, creating a routine, and taking a journey of self-discovery.

A growth mindset helps us do that. You can shape a lot of your life with your outlook on the world. We can grow our self-esteem, confidence, and leadership skills by looking for the positive side of every situation. If we let go of our toxic traits, we'll be brave and open to new opportunities.

Positive energy is contagious, too. Being open-minded and focusing on positive emotions attracts other entrepreneurs who feel the same way as you. It helps entrepreneurs adopt an entrepreneurial mindset that will help in their careers.

But for everyone, it helps us connect with people who share the same passion and goal of being authentically themselves.

We all have the ability to manifest our desires using our minds. Whether we're aware of it or not, this is an intrinsic ability in every person.

With the universal law of attraction, you can harness this power and use it for your good. This is one of the 12 laws of the universe.

It says our beliefs, thoughts, and feelings have a lot to do with what we attract. In order to attract what we want, we have to change our beliefs and thoughts.

Understanding how the law of attraction works helps speed up manifestation and make it more successful. The law of attraction is divided into 7 sub-laws.

1. Law of Manifestation

This law is one of the most popular laws of attraction. It says that whatever we focus on will manifest in our lives, no matter how good it is or how bad it is.

Our thoughts and feelings are mirrored in our surroundings, so our minds are incredibly powerful. The more positivity we try to infuse into our minds, the better our lives will be.

A decision to be conscious is always a choice. A choice to bring awareness to the present moment, a choice to recognize and prioritize what is truly meaningful, genuinely honoring, and truly value-enhancing.

On the other side, we've got to be careful about negativity creeping into our minds from time to time because that negativity will manifest negative things, which are definitely undesirable. You can achieve any of your dreams if you live a positive life.

2. The Law of Magnetism

As a result of this law, we are able to understand what has happened and what may happen in the future. It states that everything in our lives, including people, things, and circumstances, is a direct consequence of our energy vibrations.

In short, we attract what we are. It is like attracting magnets into our lives. We attract people, things, and events that share our vibrational energy.

This law can be used to accomplish what we desire in our lives. By raising our vibrations, we are able to match up to the vibration level of our desires, which results in them manifesting.

Putting this into practice is not so easy, although it seems simple enough in theory. In order to manifest our desires, we must believe in ourselves and have a burning desire to change how our minds work.

3. The Law of Harmony

A central theme of this universe is harmony. It is also an essential part of the Law of Attraction. The universe is a system of energy sources. We have to align ourselves with the flow of energy to benefit most from the universe.

Taking full advantage of the Universal energy will give us access to all the positive things that the universe has to offer. This will give us greater power for creation, more abundance, and the chance to live out our dreams.

The intention and energy you put into creating balance and aligning with the universe open the floodgates of Universal abundance, giving you access to all the wisdom, power, and blessings the world has to offer. Get in sync with yourself, with others, and with the universe.

4. The Law of Right Action

A butterfly effect is created by our actions and words. They return to us at the end. Therefore, how we behave and treat others directly impacts our own lives.

You can attract positivity and good things into your life by choosing the right path, giving a helping hand to the needy, or simply being a good person.

Even under the most challenging circumstances, you are fully capable of choosing to be good, dignified, and honorable, even when you have a natural tendency to be angry and destructive.

5. The Law of Universal Influence

Each of our actions and words has a positive impact on the world around us. Individual energy vibrations become part of the universe's vibrational frequency.

As a result of this law, we must be aware of the implications of our thoughts, emotions, actions, and words.

The universe is so intertwined that what you do will have an impact not only on your immediate family and friends but also on perfect strangers.

There are a lot of distractions that pull people away from the reality that is inside them. We are surrounded by materialism, advertisements, and all sorts of other things that pull people away from themselves.

6. The Law of Desire

A successful manifestation requires an unflinching desire, which explains why some of our desires remain unfulfilled. There is a possibility that our desire may not be strong or stable enough to withstand the rigors of manifestation.

We might think we like something, but it may not be strong and stable enough to withstand them. Unwavering desire comes from having pure intent and being free of fear, doubt, and desperation.

It's common for us to wish for different things during our lives. But when we stop to think about it, we realize most of the things we want are not important, frivolous, or detrimental to us or others.

It is important to decide whether the desire we want to manifest is something that we really want before we embark on a manifestation journey. Because only desires that are strong, steadfast, and unshakeable are likely to succeed.

7. The Law of Paradoxical Intent

As you become more eager to achieve your goal, you will push it farther away, creating the opposite of what you want.

Desperation creates the Paradox, which warns that you'll get your negative energy back if you're desperate to achieve your goals.

As a result of that repulsive vibration, it will be pushed away, turning away people and situations that could lead you to your desired outcome. You are bound to push away the very thing you are desperate for.

Gratitude can be found in the appreciation that will be rewarded with the completion of your goals, so choose to feel grateful for what you have right now. It is possible to be happy without what you want.

It's natural to become hopeful about the outcome when your desire becomes a major part of your life. In order to flow in synchronistic flow with Universal manifestation, you need to reel in any fear, urgency, or neediness, as those vibrations are both repulsive and resistant.

By valuing the future more than the present, you become attached to the result. This causes vibrations of desperation and sends out jagged waves of energy that oppose the current of abundance, removing everything you want.

When you move in the direction of frantic worry, you counter the natural flow of love and peace, which leads to more effort and disappointment.

As we have discussed before, Proponents of the law of attraction believe that your thoughts and feelings create your life. The energy you put out into the world, they say, comes back to you in what you attract.

The theory suggests that how your life pans out is ultimately within your control and that you have the power to manifest your desires using the power of positivity.

While that may seem to empower, it can also create pressure to be happy all the time. Plus, you may be wondering if there's evidence that the law of attraction theory actually works.

The catch is that the Law of Attraction can take you down a rabbit hole if you are not careful. There's a massive culture of toxic positivity that has arisen as a result of the law of attraction trend.

Some people have simplified the method to just forcing a positive mindset in any and all situations in order to manifest.

This is dangerous because it has a very real risk of invalidating people's emotional state and mental well-being. Negative feelings and low moods are valid, and they are real. You have to be able to acknowledge them first before you can have any hope of healing them.

Over time, pushing away your emotions can lead to emotional and mental health conditions. If you want to use the law of attraction, it's important to acknowledge your emotions first.

Otherwise, you run the risk of spiritually bypassing or ignoring the negative and skipping the work that real growth takes.

The process of sitting with your feelings and allowing them to exist simply can be a powerful one. From a law of attraction point of view, believers say this may release resistant energy that can prevent your desires from manifesting.

Practicing the law of attraction may make you feel pressured to be upbeat and optimistic at all times. And it is not possible to be happy all the time, and it can be damaging to your emotional health to try.

If you're using the law of attraction, it may be beneficial to explore negative emotions and use them to work through limiting beliefs and old wounds.

In the end, we're all human. We all experience the full spectrum of emotions. We must practice compassion and validate our feelings first. Once you do this, you may find yourself ready to begin manifesting your desires with a fresh perspective.

Chapter 4: Using the Law of Attraction to Lose Weight

If you're going to achieve your dreams, you might want to know what they are. Let me help you figure this out right now.

There are a lot of people who don't set goals altogether and a lot of people who don't formulate them effectively or don't review them.

When it comes to working with the Law of Attraction, this problematic approach may be what holds you back. This might be why you don't achieve success as they do.

The chances of getting the life changes you want are slim if you don't know what you want or how to express it.

Basically, if you're constantly focused on the positive, you'll attract more positive things into your life. On the other hand, if you're frequently focused on the negative, that's what you'll get.

A person's health, wealth, and relationships can be improved through the process of like energy-attracting energy, which believes that both people and thoughts are made from pure energy.

Whenever you think about something, you're constantly creating it.

You're what you think, how you feel, what you do, and what you do determines your reality, so if you want a better one, start by thinking better thoughts.

If you're clear about what you want and put those clear intentions into the universe, you'll find the resources, opportunities, and people you need to achieve your goals.

They've probably been there all along, but you didn't see them because you weren't clear about what you wanted.

Your intentional thoughts will activate the Law of Attraction, and all these resources and opportunities will show up like neon signs saying, *"Here I am! Let's do this!"*

Taking time to connect with your most authentic desires is so important at step one when setting a goal. It takes time and courage to explore what you really want in your heart, and you need time to reflect and be brave enough to confront your repressed desires.

Say you're dying to switch careers but are afraid of failing, so you hide that from yourself.

Putting aside all your assumptions about the possibility and anxiety, ask yourself:

What would I want right now if I could have anything?"

Imagining yourself having that thing is a good way to make yourself believe it's possible to achieve what you want.

Your mind turns away from the negativity associated with not having what you want when you focus on how awesome it would be to have it.

The results are that you build powerful reserves of positive energy that will propel you toward your goal. You are what you think, so what you do is what you think. Your thoughts determine your actions, and your actions announce your intentions to the universe. And the universe reacts to what you say.

Once you've figured out what you want to accomplish, it's time to fine-tune the goal-setting process. The first step is to build a deeper, more vivid picture of your goal so that you can use it as the foundation for creative visualization.

The second part it's finding the perfect words to help you express your goal, so you can create reminders and affirmations to help you get there.

Make sure you use all of your senses. That means you shouldn't just imagine yourself at your new job or wearing a cute outfit after losing weight. Instead, hear, smell, touch, and taste what it's like to get what you want.

A dream is not something you can't accomplish. So if you can imagine it, you can do it. You don't have to know every single step.

Make your mind up about what you want. Decide you deserve it. Believe you can have it, and then take one step toward it. Then another, and another.

Whenever you feel like you're not making progress toward your goals, don't beat yourself up; instead, use it as an opportunity to figure out what's holding you back.

Your success is in your hands if you set specific goals, visualize them every day, and self-monitor to keep your mind on track.

There's no limit to what this law works with. It's not just people or energy; it works with stuff too. You'll get it, no matter what you want, whether it's money, a new car, a new house, a new toy, or a new video game. All you have to do is ask, believe, and receive.

In summary, what you think becomes a reality. If you believe that you're fat, then you are. If you think you won't lose weight, then you won't.

The universe will send you the exact vibration you give it. If you think you won't lose weight because of your thoughts, then you won't lose weight unless you change your thoughts.

The Internet is full of people who have lost hundreds of pounds that you can see. There's no new information about weight loss.

The biggest change came from the way people thought about their weight loss journey. Instead of thinking, I can't do it, they thought I can,

Thinking along the lines of, "I've decided, and it'll happen."

The Law of Attraction can really speed up the weight loss process, even though it's unrealistic.

Positivity can be the key to finally creating an entirely new path for yourself if you've tried a bunch of fad diets, aggravating exercise plans, and failed weight loss commitments.

If you think about it like this, your thoughts and actions coming into alignment result in inspired action that reflects a specific intention. In this case, it's losing weight.

Our cognitive and emotional lives are entirely at odds with our outward commitments to lose weight because of underlying negative feelings and unhelpful assumptions.

It's a lot about looking inside and changing your relationship with food, exercise, and body image to manifest long-lasting weight loss.

In addition, using the Law of Attraction for weight loss will boost your overall health. As a result, you'll have a new set of tools to help you achieve your goals.

A powerful way to take control of your weight is to start seeing yourself as active. For instance, if you're looking to lose weight, you should develop more self-awareness.

Research shows that if you believe you're doing more physical activity than the average person if you're more likely to lose weight, even if you don't change anything else about your daily routine, you're more likely to lose fat.

Let's say you want to lose weight, but you don't know how.

Take a look at what you're gonna eat and think about it before you do it - If you're trying to lose weight, you need to eat right and smart.

Keep track of how many calories you eat or count them if you need to. Don't eat out or order online if you only make your meal ahead of time.

You'll be able to lose weight if you eat foods of many different colors instead of just junk food. Look for foods of many different colors. Eating a rainbow diet has many health benefits and can also trick your brain.

Sleeping well will solve half of your health problems. A good night's sleep will make you feel good when you wake up. You should sleep at least eight hours per night if you eat a lot at night.

If you put your mind to it, you can lose weight. You've been creating your present weight the whole time you've been alive. You need to shift your focus and energy to see positive results in the weight loss area.

Your thinking and beliefs now won't be the same as your thinking and beliefs in the future. You gotta transform yourself from the inside out to truly transform.

Is the law of attraction really effective at losing weight?

In order to get the body you want, you have to change the way you see yourself. It all starts with getting your priorities straight. Weight loss is impossible if you're not in alignment.

Your underlying assumptions determine your vibrational frequency. My vibration represents the way I see myself and how I feel about myself.

Affirmations help you believe in your dreams and make you more confident in your abilities. When you say out loud what your dreams, goals, and ambitions are, you immediately eliminate doubts and feel more confident about yourself.

You can be sure that the things you say become true, and you can handle any problem that comes your way with affirmations.

It may sound too simple and unpretentious to be of any use, but you'd be wrong. These positive statements are important to raise your self-confidence and self-esteem.

You gotta affirm, but don't forget to do it too. Take action because nothing happens without it. Wishing for something and waiting for it to show up isn't how manifestation works. In order to make it happen, you have to put in all the effort, and the universe will do its part at the right time.

Losing weight involves watching what you eat and what you don't eat. Working out regularly is important. You need a healthy lifestyle.

In order for your actions to work, you have to believe they'll come through. That's why faith in the universe is so essential to manifesting. In the hope that the universe will support your effort to change your mindset and lose weight, you put in the effort to change your mindset and lose weight.

Your manifestation attempt will fail if you don't believe the universe is on your side. If you don't believe the universe is on your side, your manifestation effort will fail.

You should also be careful not to become obsessed with the desire. You should learn to let it go and not let it consume you. You have to find the right balance between focusing on it and obsessing over it.

Keeping positive and avoiding negative thoughts can help you lose weight. It's the same approach for manifesting anything you want.

Manifesting is easier said than done. It's easy to read about and understand but hard to follow. If it's your first time manifesting, be gentle with yourself and be kind to yourself when you make mistakes. Getting used to manifestation methods and techniques takes time.

If you use the law of attraction to lose weight, it's a powerful tool. To reach your target weight, you have to focus on your goals, visualize yourself at your ideal weight, and take action steps towards those goals. The law of attraction will work with you.

The Law of Attraction says you attract what you focus on and feel passionate about into your life.

Putting your focus on the good and positive things in your life will automatically attract more of them. And focusing on lack and negativity will bring more of it into your life. That's how it works.

When you understand how the Law of Attraction works, you can change your results and create a better life consciously and intentionally.

The situations you encounter during your day can start to feel different if you choose to respond differently. Instead of focusing on things that make you angry, focus on things that make you happy.

And you can choose to create the future you want simply by intentionally taking the time to focus on what you want your life to look and feel like – instead of unconsciously living life by default, often creating the exact opposite of what you want.

The fact is, you are constantly creating your own reality at every moment.

Your thoughts determine your feelings, your feelings determine your actions, and your actions determine your reality – so if you want to create a better reality, you have to start by thinking better thoughts.

Because when you are clear about what you want, and you put those clear intentions out into the universe, the resources, the people, and the opportunities you need to achieve your goals will start appearing to you, almost like magic.

Chances are they were there all along, but because you weren't clear on what you wanted, you never noticed them.

With the power of focus, you conserve your energies and do not dissipate them on irrelevant thoughts or activities. This is why developing concentration is vital for anyone aspiring to be more efficient and take charge of his or her life.

This skill is essential for every kind of success. Without it, you scatter your energy and waste time, but you can accomplish great things with it.

By taking the time to focus on what you want your life to look and feel like, you'll be able to create the future you want instead of unconsciously living life by default, creating the opposite.

Whenever you think about something, you're constantly creating it.

In order to create a better reality, you've got to think of better thoughts first. Your thoughts determine your feelings, your feelings determine your actions, and your actions determine your reality.

It's almost like magic when you're clear about what you want and put those clear intentions out into the universe, and then you start getting the resources, people, and opportunities you need.

They've probably been there all along, but you didn't see them because you weren't clear about what you wanted.

Focus conserves energy, so you don't waste it on useless thoughts or activities. That's why developing concentration is essential for anyone looking to be more efficient and more in charge of their lives.

Without it, you'll scatter your energy and waste time, but with it, you'll be able to accomplish amazing things. If your gut feelings point towards a desire to refrain from taking certain actions, you will feel apprehension, and apprehension will arrive suddenly.

It is important to differentiate between urgent calls from your inner being for discontinuance and excitement. It is okay to feel uneasy when preparing to experience a new experience, but don't let your interpretation of what you are experiencing stop you from doing so.

Better still, allow yourself to take a few moments to breathe deeply and welcome and appreciate the challenge ahead of you.

It can be pleasurable rather than nerve-wracking to extend yourself when you are aware that uncomfortable feelings are a sign that you are doing so.

Chapter 5: Food is My Friend

"How can we ever know what we're truly capable of if we're not trying to do what we don't think we can spend every single day? And that means being afraid and doing it anyway." – Siri Lindley

In our brains, we crave comfort. It's all too easy to binge-watch Netflix instead of working out or sticking to what you know instead of learning something new.

In order to truly grow, we must learn to get comfortable with being uncomfortable – and without growth, we can never truly be happy.

Sure, you're going to be scared of failing, you're going to be scared of being rejected, but you've got to try.

There's more to being comfortable with being uncomfortable than just athletes – it can help you in your career, your relationships, and your personal life.

Find out what's making you uncomfortable, embrace what's going on, reframe the experience positively – and repeat until you're okay with discomfort.

"I'm okay."

The most common phrase I hear is "I'm doing fine" because most of us are not necessarily happy, sad, or angry. In my own life, I tend to think of being okay as being content, maybe a little bored, or just at peace.

People usually start off in this category, feeling angry, hurt, sad, anxious, confused, and many more emotions. But good, okay, and bad are bad ways to describe our emotions.

We don't like to experience uncomfortable emotions. Those might be the "bad" feelings like embarrassment, guilt, shame, and hurt.

If you label them as bad, you tend to judge them and don't want to explore them when you do feel them. So we push them away, minimize them, and find other ways to escape.

When you start labeling your emotions as comfortable or uncomfortable, you can discover what they're saying to you. Emotions are like a compass to me. Any feeling you feel is trying to tell you what to do. Happiness tells you you should keep going, while guilt tells you you are doing something wrong.

Your comfortable and uncomfortable emotions might surprise you. Some people are uncomfortable feeling some emotions that others might find comfortable, like feeling shame and guilt or not feeling joy. It takes time to build emotional language and awareness before you can dive deep into emotions.

Whether it is an irksome sensation or an unpleasant experience, all of these things cause us a sense of discomfort, whether it is an embarrassing conversation or a mosquito bite. In general, we define "discomfort" as the absence of comfort, but it is unclear which came first.

A diseased body is one that is not functioning properly, or more accurately, one that is not working according to the laws of nature.

It is only when a body is out of harmony, out of harmony with what it should be doing, that it manifests disease. This state of disharmony has no symptoms at first.

Depending on who we are, we all have a threshold for being at dis-ease. The higher that threshold, the more comfortable we are with being uncomfortable.

It is, however, possible to take steps to help you step out of your comfort zone more easily, regardless of your level of comfort.

Feeling dis-ease is normal and healthy for everyone, so don't be scared to be uncomfortable. When faced with something new or different, most people experience some degree of discomfort at first, but they usually adjust to the situation once they get used to it.

This feeling of dis-ease is something that you have to overcome at some point in your life. If you want to grow personally, you must embrace discomfort.

The first step is to identify what makes you uncomfortable and how they make you feel. By understanding the triggers that make you uncomfortable and facing those challenges rather than turning away from them, you will be able to identify what experiences to pursue.

The idea of naming this grief is powerful. It helps us feel what is inside of us. Several of my coworkers have told me in the past week that they were having a hard time or that they cried last night.

When you name it, you feel it, and it flows through you. Emotions require motion. We must acknowledge what we experience. The self-help movement has led to the unfortunate byproduct that we are the first generation to be able to talk about our emotions.

When we feel sad, we tell ourselves, "I shouldn't feel that; other people have worse problems." We can — we should — stop at the first feeling. I feel sad. Let me spend five minutes feeling sad.

Feeling your sadness, fear, and anger, regardless of whether or not anyone else feels them is your work. It doesn't help to fight it because your body is producing it. By allowing the feelings to happen, they'll happen in an orderly way, which empowers us. Then we aren't victims.

In an orderly way?

The truth is that we sometimes try to avoid feeling what we feel because we have this idea of a "gang of feelings." If I let in sadness, the gang of bad feelings will take over me.

This means that we have feelings that move through us. We feel them, they go, and then we move on to the next. There is no gang out there to get us. Let yourself feel the grief and keep going.

Believing in yourself and those around you is the key to success. Without self-confidence, one will never do anything.

You cannot hope for a better tomorrow if you lack belief in your abilities. You will not complete your work to the best of your ability if you begin to doubt yourself.

The loss of hope will engulf your life in sorrow and darkness, but eventually, the light will return, and you will be able to live your life to the fullest. Life will never be perfect, but you have to do the best with what you've got.

The feeling of dis-ease and making mistakes is one thing, but at some point, you should forgive yourself and move on. Otherwise, you will only hold yourself back and prevent yourself from taking risks and achieving your goals.

It's ultimately down to you to believe in yourself since this will take you one step closer to manifesting a better life.

You can only live a happy and productive life if you believe in yourself. When one is completely confident in oneself, they are capable of doing anything one sets their mind to without fear of failure.

Because of this, many self-confident people are successful in anything they do. Through their general handling of life, they also inspire us. There are, unfortunately, many people who lack confidence in themselves.

As a result, they are faced with many challenges in life, from effective communication with other people to how they present themselves to others.

A person can accomplish anything if they have a positive mindset. Life will always be a roller coaster ride with many ups and downs. Encouragement boosts confidence. What counts is how you apply it in life.

"To be yourself in a world that is constantly trying to make you something else is the greatest accomplishment." ~ **Ralph Waldo Emerson**

It is natural for each of us to have things we love. These things are both deeply enjoyable, and they are aligned with what we want to become. When we are doing these things, we feel both fun and joy in the present, yet at the same time, we feel content with the person we want to become.

As well as things we like, there are things we merely do for pleasure. These things may provide momentary blips of joy, but they don't really improve our self-esteem or make us feel fulfilled in any way.

There is a simple way to dramatically increase your level of happiness in your everyday life as well as your long-term fulfillment with who you are and where you are in your life: Do more of the things you love.

A person's happiness is largely determined by their passion for what they do. More than money, fame, or status, passion is something almost completely under their control. Your career, relationships, or health may be thrown around by outside forces, but what they love is largely up to them.

You can't avoid the things you have to do, but you won't be able to avoid them. The things you have to do will take up a lot of time, sometimes even all of it.

You need to work on removing the things you have to do and replacing them with the things you love to do in order to become more successful, but even the most successful people will never be completely free of this.

There may not be a way for you to excuse things you need to do, but you can certainly make adjustments to the things you like or reduce guilt regarding the things you feel you should do.

To enhance these feelings, you can raise vibrations in your home to make it a better place to live, sleep, and enjoy your free time. Living in your home should make you happy, positive, and safe. Using these vibrations, you'll remove the negative energy from your home and let in new, positive energy.

When you clean your energy, you automatically raise your internal vibration to a higher level. This will lead to you feeling lighter, happier, and more peaceful as a result.

Keeping your vibrations up and positive can be accomplished by doing just a few simple things—and the same applies to making changes to your surroundings.

Positive vibrations exude happiness and promote good health. Getting rid of negativity and negative energy from your environment will help you feel more relaxed. The higher your vibration, the lower your stress levels.

Our desire to manifest must be aligned with the higher vibration that we are trying to achieve.

The more low vibrational activities we engage in, the lower our vibration and the less likely we are to realize our dreams and desires.

Obviously, we can't be high vibe all the time, nor should we want to - we all go through ups and downs!

It is in this state that we are able to attract great things, but we want to generally maintain a positive vibration.

It is possible to become more conscious of your daily habits once you begin to raise your vibration and begin to live in alignment with what you wish to attract once you learn how to raise your vibration.

In engaging in thoughts, feelings, or behaviors of a higher vibration, we naturally begin to resonate with the same vibration.

You need to understand that our feelings are not all negative. There's something flowing strongly within us that needs to be embraced. If we can turn and go along with our feelings, we will be able to achieve our goals.

It can be extremely difficult to feel powerless and self-conscious when dealing with weight and body issues. Losing weight is the top New Year's Eve resolution in America because it is such a common issue! Weight loss is the most common resolution, so people want to lose weight, but they don't know where to begin.

Many people feel that losing weight will boost their self-esteem, improve their stamina, and improve their overall health.

Some feel that losing weight will make shopping for clothing easier, and they will enjoy how the clothing fits. Because they are self-conscious or too out of shape, others feel that their weight prevents them from engaging in certain activities.

People eat a lot more than you do. But you see slender people eating a lot more than you do who have the body condition that they desire. That's because of metabolism. Energy balance in your body determines how your body looks and feels.

It doesn't matter how much you do if you're vibrationally upstream. The results won't come if you're vibrationally upstream. That's why your metabolism slows down. That's why you hold on to unhealthy habits.

You are always fighting that vibrational tug of war whenever you experience heart disease, stroke, or any dis-ease or sickness. That's why every disease, illness, and ailment is always related to vibrations pointed upward.

The majority of people who want to lose weight feel as if they've tried everything. They've tried diets, tried weight-loss shakes, taken weight-loss pills, or jumped into the gym hard.

You wondered if you were always destined to be this size because you didn't manage to lose all the weight, and once you did, it popped right back on. You wonder if you will always be this size.

Basically, you're balancing your vibrations, so you do things with ease. Your resistance begins to dissolve, and therefore, more ideas start flowing to you.

As the weight begins to fall off, your energy increases, you want to move more, and you decide to get on the scale for the first time in several days, only to be pleasantly surprised by the results.

In order to improve vibration, you should use action, which is a human technique. After all, we typically hear people tell us to clean up our vibrations and carry out inspired actions in order to improve our vibration.

You fall in love with yourself when you apply actions that improve your feelings, and the improvement increases your energy and inspires you to do more. The cycle goes on until you feel motivated from the inside, and inspiration comes from within.

Whenever you feel uncomfortable with your body, whether it's how it moves, looks, or feels, your standards increase. The unhappier you are with your body, the higher your standards will be.

It is important for you to learn how to shift your vibration so that your body can become the way you desire when you shift it.

Once you understand how vibrations can help you lose weight, it's time to get started and believe in your abilities.

Ascertain that you will give yourself as much time as you need to accomplish your goals. You must start new patterns of energy and practice so that you can achieve long-term results.

Chapter 6: Controlling Your Thoughts

The road to success is full of twists and turns.

Every human being has to overcome every obstacle in the way. Hard work is an essential requirement. Humanity cannot achieve success in a short time frame.

I've always been told to work hard and to be successful by my parents and that I should become a good person in order to be successful.

Sometimes, success feels confusing to me.

There are proverbs that propagate the same vague ideas.

No pain, no gain.

Hard work never goes to waste.

Success comes to you sooner or later.

The media promotes the narrative that hard work will lead to success. If you work hard, you'll find a way to rise above terrible situations and get what you deserve.

You're successful because you've worked hard, so success is a demonstration of your virtue.

The sad thing is that it doesn't always happen.

I've seen many deserving classmates get unexpectedly poor results. Moreover, the poor who struggle with diligence every day get trapped in a vicious cycle that's hard to break out of. Even though I worked hard for my A level, I still screwed up a lot.

Right away, you're burning with guilt over what you've missed; you're wondering if there's something you've done wrong that caused your world to collapse.

The worst part is when you've genuinely put in the effort; you wonder if you've actually lazily done it after all.

When you look back on things, you feel like you have done everything you could. Does that mean you're incompetent - that even your best isn't enough?

Your feelings aren't just disappointment; they're shame and indignation because you feel the whole world is judging you for seemingly being "lazy, profligate," and therefore not worthy.

As well as feeling robbed of your destiny, it may make you feel like life is laughing at the fast one it pulled on you after you sacrificed everything and put everything on the line. You feel cold scorn and judgment from those around you now instead of sympathy for all the wasted time and effort you wasted.

Because of the pernicious entitlement mentality, thinking success comes solely from hard work; as if hard work alone could guarantee success. But it doesn't work that way, and success is also determined by chance.

Even so, society is structurally designed to assume differently, creating subconscious assumptions about every failure. This type of cruel mentality causes a lot of people to feel scorned.

We've all been in a situation where we worked hard and failed to land a new job or a key promotion simply because we didn't work hard enough.

Over the years, we have been told that *"Just work hard, and things will work out for you,"* This is actually half the truth.

Working hard is one of the most important ingredients for success, but it's risky to think that's all you need.

Working hard isn't enough anymore. In today's world, hard work isn't enough for success. There's more to it than that.

People who succeed work hard but smart and differently. They make an impact, are creative, and are different from their competitors.

People think the repetition of any task brings mastery, but that's not true. Mastery comes from continuous practice and learning from mistakes while constantly improving your approach.

Almost everyone wants to get successful, but very few do. Why? Since it takes a lot of patience, hard work, sacrifices, and, most importantly, perseverance or self-determination.

Many people commit a common mistake when trying to achieve their goals: procrastinating. They say they'd like to do things, but they don't.

There's no denying that everyone wants success, but only a few actually get it. Why? Because it takes hard work, sacrifice, patience, and, most importantly, perseverance.

It's a common mistake people make when they're striving to achieve their goals, and that's procrastinating. They say they're going to do it, but they don't.

"Beyond mountains are more mountains."

It's the ones who can overcome obstacles that will succeed because obstacles never cease, and people don't give up too soon when they encounter rejections and failures. People give up way too soon after rejections and failures. The ones who succeed are persistent in following through on their dreams 'till they get there.

People who work unreasonably long hours are so consumed by their jobs that they can't see the opportunities that are right in front of them.

In order to keep up the momentum, it's essential to take breaks in between. These breaks will replenish your energy so you can keep going.

It takes a lot of hard work, courage, determination, and dedication to reach your goals. Just follow your dream, get obsessed with it, and make it happen.

In the end, hard work is honorable. It makes a person respect themselves and others. It's all in my mind.

The way you think about yourself and the world around you can have a radical impact on how your life turns out. The way you think about yourself and the world around you can have a huge impact on learning, managing stress, creating success, and even your immune system.

Understanding both abundance and scarcity mindsets will help you discover where you fit on the spectrum.

It can be helpful to cultivate mindfulness to figure out whether your thoughts are creating a mindset of scarcity or abundance. By taking notice of the kinds of thoughts that are circling in your head, you can begin to shift those thoughts.

The enemy of abundance is contracted awareness. A study found that people aren't noticing other possibilities right in front of them because they're focused on one thing. When you think about abundance, you need to loosen up your mind and expand your awareness.

To believe in yourself, you should understand and build confidence in what you are great at and enjoy doing.

You'll learn how to share your gifts and help people who can benefit from your knowledge. Start a personal brand presence online or in person so you can confidently share what you do.

We're surrounded by abundance because existence is infinite. There's nothing that can't exist in an infinite universe, like lack. Just look at this planet. There are people, animals, insects, and all kinds of creatures.

Aside from that, there's a lot of food in crops, plants, fruit, and vegetables. Everything nourishes the whole, like the sun that shines each day, the rain that moistens the soil and provides us with water to drink, the air we breathe, and the trees we plant. Everything nourishes and provides.

When the universe is infinite, everything should already be available to us. Everything should be readily available inside of us. So, abundance is life itself, the manifestation of existence.

Apparently, the universe is always expanding and growing, and new stars are being created.

Plentitude is everywhere in the universe, but it can also show up in your personal life if you let it.

In abundance, you'll find trees, plants, animals, and various forms of life, plus stars and universes that are unending.

A star is born every hour, a tree grows every year, a person is born every day, and an energy source is discovered every day.

The abundance mindset believes there are enough resources for everyone in the world - and to be grateful for everything the universe gives us.

In contrast, a scarcity mindset believes that the world's resources are finite. When someone gets something, everyone loses something.

We know that what we believe in our minds leads to our actions, resulting in our reality. But belief isn't something you can prove.

We can manifest our beliefs into reality when we exert our life force energy, so in essence, what we believe becomes real for us, even if it's an illusion, since believing in lack is basically saying there is no life.

This is a contradiction. There is only life. Death is not the opposite of life. Birth is the opposite of death. So, all there is life. And abundance is just another word for life.

If you pause and look right now, billions of cells work together in harmony to support you. It's not about BELIEVING in abundance; it's about recognizing it.

A trillion chemical reactions keep you healthy. Your body is made up of molecules dancing! You are the expression of creation. So, if this is true, then there is no lack except in what you think about.

Our society still downplays luck, putting more emphasis on hard work and aptitude rather than recognizing the importance of luck. Income inequality has intensified the debate.

There's a lot of fortune involved in success, and individuals contribute a bit to their own success, so their success probably involves more than just themselves.

If you've done well in the past, go ahead and learn from it, but don't forget to think about the present as a completely new set of circumstances that probably contributed to your success in the past. Taking shortcuts won't help you get your own hot hand.

In addition to luck, sometimes favoritism plays a big role in people's lives. Favoritism can either bring success or hurt people when it's turned into harassment.

It's been proven that people's brains work the same way when they feel excluded as when they are hurt.

It's important that people outside the inner circle don't feel unappreciated and excluded, which leads to disengagement and disillusionment.

Team spirit is also damaged as a result of this kind of management style, which has a negative impact on productivity and ultimately means employees are more likely to leave.

The ability to adopt a positive mental attitude can have a substantial impact on your success, regardless of what negativity surrounds you.

The act of working towards positive thoughts in your everyday interactions with yourself and others can help you develop greater self-confidence, strengthen your relationships, and achieve what you want in life.

If you have a negative mindset, you will overthink your interactions, your work, and your efforts, and you will believe that none of it is sufficient. A negative mindset can also make you comfortable with failure, which is certainly not going to help you.

When you are negative, you cannot see the forest for the trees. It narrows your thoughts, stressing you out and making you react negatively.

When you see only one problem at a time, you do not have room to consider alternative solutions. When you learn to counter negativity with positive thoughts, your career trajectory will continue upward.

Positivity doesn't come naturally to many people; it requires a conscious effort on the part of the individual to rewire their brains to think positively.

The more you work towards a positive mindset, the more joy, contentment, and love you'll find.

You can get a big boost from positive thinking when you think positively. In a similar fashion to a downward spiral, which is associated with the slippery slope of negative thoughts, a positive spiral can give you the momentum you need to broaden your horizons and get more successful. Make sure you use the baby steps tactic you've learned about to keep yourself on track.

A positive attitude also helps you deal with feedback and conflict in a new way. For example, if you get constructive criticism that makes you squirm, you can use it as a learning tool.

You can do the same for conflict: you can build new pathways in your brain to deal with further setbacks or problems so you can handle conflicts well.

The power of positive thinking is behind all success, even though most people think it comes down to work ethic, persistence, and drive.

Make positive changes to your thinking so you'll believe in yourself and be successful. You'll be surprised how much better you'll feel when you think positively.

It affects all aspects of your life because the limiting beliefs say you can't improve your circumstances, earn enough money, or even make life better in general.

Most times, people visualize situations that are not real. They put together negative images in their heads and live life worrying about perceived scarcity.

You feel every goal is out of reach if you have a scarcity mindset. Because you believe there is never enough of anything, be it time, money, affection, or relationships, you can't bring out your best.

A scarcity mindset makes people wonder if they're going to miss out on life's good things and if time is running out.

Make a conscious effort to think positive and happy thoughts to get rid of the scarcity mindset.

By reassuring yourself that everything will work out, you'll be able to live the life of your dreams. You'll be able to soothe anxiety and look forward to the possibilities of growth, evolution, and taking yourself to the next level of success and happiness.

You're not what you lack, so think about what you do have, what's going right in your life, and the awesome people you're surrounded by.

Being grateful for what you have will help you appreciate the good things in your life and help you develop an abundance mindset.

Your mindset determines your life trajectory. If you want to flourish in life, you need to take advantage of the power of positive thinking.

Having an open mind and a willingness to better your life will give you plenty of resources and endless opportunities. So let go of scarcity, embrace abundance, and get work done. That's the quickest way to live the life of your dreams and achieve massive success.

The mole in Positive Thinking is the negative thoughts that pop up from time to time. As hard as it may sound, you'll get used to it when you see how easy it is to manifest what you want.

Creating opportunities for your positive thoughts, expecting them, and looking for signs that they have manifested is the next step. You've got to stay consistent. You're the one who's going to make things happen.

Think about what you want to accomplish and create opportunities that match your goals. For example, if you want a promotion, you should take courses that will help you get it.

When you live intentionally, know what you want, and get it, you'll have a better, less anxious, and more fulfilled life. Positive thinking comes from knowing what you want and getting it.

Chapter 7: Power of Visualization

Visualization involves utilizing the brain's capabilities to achieve your goals and bringing ideas from "platonic heaven" to reality.

Though visualization has been around for a long time, it's becoming more popular now that people are focusing more on mindfulness and positive thinking.

There's beauty to visualization because it's something you can learn, not something you have to do every day. All it takes is commitment.

It's awesome to visualize your life and achieve amazing things. It's hard to accomplish your goals and objectives if you don't understand the power of visualization and how to use the tools and techniques to visualize.

It's important that you understand the power of visualization in this regard. You gotta visualize achieving your success.

As the saying goes, a battle is won twice—first in your head and then in reality. You'll have a mental script first and a real script later. If you visualize yourself well, you can become the person you want to be.

In fact, your mind churns out thoughts all the time, whether you like it or not. When you visualize, the internal chatter slowly disappears, and your brain slowly becomes calm.

Getting rid of clutter and getting clarity on your thoughts is the first step to becoming successful.

Researchers have found that people who visualize have a higher chance of building habits and succeeding.

The purpose of visualization is to help you "rewire" your brain and change your habits. It reorients your conscious and subconscious thoughts, and it helps you get rid of bad habits.

Distractions are gone, your concentration is enhanced, your subconscious mind is stronger, your dreams become bigger, you become more motivated, and you develop an internal locus of control.

Getting your physical print and mental print aligned will help you align your outside world with your inside world.

The best visionaries harness the power of visualization, inspire collaboration and teamwork, and make their vision a reality.

"First, have a definite, clear, practical ideal; a goal, an objective. Second, have the necessary means to achieve your ends; wisdom, money, materials, and methods. Third, adjust all your means to that end."

-Aristotle

With visualization, you can achieve your desired outcomes simply by focusing on positive mental images. It's a time-tested, proven way to get what you want.

The power of visualization comes from the fact that it impacts our subconscious minds, and without even knowing it, we are moving in the direction of our thoughts.

People around the world use visualization on a daily basis to get where they want to go, personally and professionally.

It's hard to define the power of visualization, but at its most basic level, it's seeing your goals as though they're already done.

It's about understanding how your subconscious mind works. By visualizing something, you're imprinting it there.

In the midst of a conflict between your conscious mind and the current reality, where your mind works, there will be a conflict.

Reality and your vision aren't different in the subconscious mind. It just wants to minimize conflicts.

Think of your subconscious mind as your inner collaborator that aligns your conscious and subconscious minds.

When you visualize something, you see what you need to do to achieve it, and you're attracted to those things, which will help you accomplish what you've set out to do.

You'll hear about visualization and the Law of Attraction, where positive or negative thoughts bring about something.

Most people believe that people and their thoughts are made up of "pure energy" and that the energy of your thoughts is connected to everything.

The power of positive thinking rests on the premise that your thoughts attract like energy.

Practicing visualization regularly is like practicing meditation.

With repeated practice, the mind doesn't know what's real from what's not, especially when you incorporate all five senses.

By tricking the brain, you can make it think you've already got what you want or that you've already worked out the kinks to a problem, like more confidence or better grades.

Simply put, visualization is a motivator that might lead to successful behavior changes.

When elite athletes visualize worst-case scenarios, they prepare for real-life situations by imagining falling, having pain, dealing with equipment malfunctions, and the like.

Basically, their brains have already dealt with the scenario, so they don't have to worry about handling it during a competition.

The power of visualization might seem a little skeptical to you if you're a very literal or pragmatic person.

Many don't disagree that visualizing success is often just a lazy substitute for actually making it happen.

In reality, visualization involves much more than just sitting back and imagining that great things will happen. Lots of research suggests that mental imagery can have a huge impact on how we act.

A common misconception about visualization is that all you have to do is visualize, and things will appear in your life.

Using visualization to show up as the best version of ourselves needs to go beyond visualization.

Visualization is based on neuroscience, which explains how the brain works.

Using our brains more effectively in a structured, practical way can seem like magic when combined with vision and strategic action.

Seeing stuff in your mind's eye isn't just about the mind. When we visualize, especially if we've created a scene in our head, we use the right brain.

By integrating the rational, analytical, verbal, and intuitive parts of the brain, we tap into more creative, intuitive, and holistic parts.

By visualizing, we activate more of ourselves and our capacity. Visualizing is powerful.

It doesn't just activate more right brain areas. It doesn't just tap into underused parts of the brain.

Connecting the left brain's analytical functions with the right brain's creativity, intuition, and inner peace levels our brain's functionality.

Integration means that when we visualize, our brains are working together, creating a more powerful effect and increasing our productivity.

That way, we can show up as our best selves and achieve what we want, one day at a time.

When we visualize, our brain reacts as if it were happening in real life. It's like we live multiple lives.

Our subconscious mind reacts as if we're currently experiencing a success scene from our past or practicing a perfect performance in the future.

Our subconscious mind doesn't know the difference, so visualizers can train it to show up as their best selves in any situation.

It's like being in a giant quantum sea full of vibrational energy whose waves are responsive to our thoughts. Our thoughts are constantly expressing themselves in our lives. Once we realize this, we can start designing our lives with clarity and purpose.

Visualizing is all about seeing yourself already having what you want. It's a mental trick to make it work.

Live as if it's happening right now, rather than hoping you'll get there or building confidence that it will one day happen.

There's a part of you that knows it's just a trick, but the subconscious mind doesn't know the difference between real and imagined.

Whatever images you create in your head, your subconscious will act on them, no matter what reality you're living in.

A daily practice of visualizing your dreams will accelerate them into reality.

See it, feel it, believe it.

"Your imagination is your preview of life's coming attractions."

-Albert Einstein

There's good news, the conscious mind can only think one thing at a time, and you get to decide what that thought is.

Rather than visualizing what you don't want, imagine what you do want.

When you regularly practice visualization, you'll inevitably gravitate toward your dominant thoughts and feel the resulting emotion, no matter how positive or negative they are.

You'd be amazed at how easy it is to relax with a few minutes of visualization. The subconscious doesn't know the difference between imagination and reality, so it believes whatever we put on paper.

Imagination can trick our subconscious into believing things that aren't true and evoke specific emotions and feelings.

By visualizing calming pictures, you're letting your mind release what it holds, like a muscle. If you visualize calming pictures, you're letting your mind relax.

Visualizations can become your happy place when you close your eyes and begin to visualize. It's like sending your brain a message that it's time to let go of anything you've been mentally squeezing, like worries and fears.

The power of visualization can be used for a lot of things, like grounding yourself with pictures and scenarios.

Manifesting your desires into reality is another way to visualize. Being able to form a clear mental picture of what you want is one of the most powerful things we can do.

Getting your goals accomplished through visualization is supported by three mental laws.

Regardless of what you believe, with feeling, you become what you believe. You are the culmination of all your beliefs.

Your beliefs are true for you no matter what they say, even if they're not consistent with reality.

There's so much power in our minds that even if we believe and visualize something based on false information, it still affects us either positively or negatively.

Whatever self-limiting beliefs we believe, they'll become true as long as we believe them.

"Whatever you can conceive and believe, you can achieve."

-Napoleon Hill

You can't imagine something without the power to make it come true. However, this doesn't mean you don't have lessons to learn, obstacles to overcome, or hardships to endure before your desires become a reality.

To make your dreams come true, you have to be willing to pay for them. Visualizing your goals is a major step.

This concept of self-fulfillment has been extensively researched and supports the notion that what you expect becomes true.

People who have high levels of accomplishments talk to themselves all the time like they expect great things.

Negative thoughts and visualizations are also common among unhappy people.

It's like we're living magnets - we radiate thought energy and attract people and things that resonate with our dominant thoughts and mental images.

You've got to change your thoughts and visualizations if you want to attract different people and circumstances.

The Universe works by law, not chance. You can improve your life by manufacturing the beliefs and expectations you want.

Usually, when people talk about visualization, they mean visualizing that you have effortlessly reached your goal and are enjoying the result, as inspired by the law of attraction concept. That's not what I mean by visualization.

The best way to overcome excuses, resistance, failures, and other challenges on your way is to visualize how you're going to go through it.

Seeing just the end result drains your motivation because your brain cools down, thinking it's all done and doesn't have the energy for the hard work.

In Mindful Self-Discipline, visualization is about practicing perseverance. Visualization helps you visualize yourself doing the action, facing obstacles, then getting over them.

When you visualize success, you probably picture conflicts, misunderstandings, and fights with your partner.

Imagination yourself finding the tools, the clarity, and the energy to successfully work through the storm, coming out of it stronger and more united.

It's a lot more realistic and practical than just visualizing eternal honeymoon moments.

Visualize everything as vividly as you can, as if you were actually there. If you're not good at visualizing, just imagine how your mind works.

You really want to make it real and experience it firsthand so that you prime your brain for new behavior.

There's no doubt that visualization is important. The world has gotten way too complicated—from climate change to wholesale business transformation—and the challenges we face are huge.

Our mental models aren't up to the task of thinking about them because they're interconnected, fluid, and ambiguous.

With visualization, we're able to offload these cognitive tasks to a physical space where we can work systematically.

The fact that we use visual information differently than auditory or other perceptual data is no surprise. Our brains devote 80% of their energy to visual information.

As a matter of fact, visual stimuli can be distributed to 35 different areas of the brain, so they can be processed in parallel.

What makes for a good visualization?

First, it should accentuate what's important in a situation and deemphasize what's not. When looking at visualization, you should be able to pick up on the most salient points right from the start.

Second, it should be understandable and clear. And finally, it should be capable of being manipulated, i.e., it should allow people to engage with it in some way.

A good visualization should lead people to an "a-ha" moment—to find their way from the current state to a desired future state.

When visualizing a problem, start by thinking through the various audiences and challenges involved—both in the current state and a desired future state.

Then you can "make a scene" by visualizing different elements of the situation, using nodes for the people involved, links to capture their connections and relationships, and territories to express areas of meaning.

Visualizing or externalizing the situation can help you think through the problem more clearly. You may begin to see differences in the roles played by various individuals and understand the dynamics of their interactions more clearly.

By doing this, you'll be able to add detail and see the nuance that wasn't evident at the start. Think of it as turning thoughts into images so you can bring something more analytical and critical to the challenge. And the more you do it, the easier it gets.

Other than that, there's only one mental requirement: to eliminate our tendency to try and figure everything out in our heads.

Think about it and sketch it out on a whiteboard or flip chart. Don't worry about how it looks.

Success here doesn't measure artistic value. It's about the visualization's ability to help you think through problems, communicate and collaborate with your team, and, ultimately, come up with a solution that moves your organization or business forward.

Creative visualization can help you lose weight. When you visualize your body looking how you want it to, your subconscious mind shapes it to match your image.

Visualizing in accordance with the laws of visualization won't instantly change your body shape. But it will improve how you look, help you lose weight, and make you feel better.

The image of your dream body will ingrain itself into your subconscious, motivating you to change.

In turn, your subconscious mind will shape your body based on your mental image of yourself. But you have to also eat well and exercise.

Eating well and exercising are essential for losing weight, but with the help of creative visualization, this process can become faster and more pleasant.

The kind of thoughts and emotions you think and feel has an impact on your body, for better or worse.

Negative thinking, stress, fear, worries, and anger hurt the body. Under these conditions, the body releases toxins into the blood, which affect it adversely.

On the other hand, positive thinking, happiness, love, and confidence heal, strengthen and energize the body.

When losing weight, don't see yourself disgusted with certain foods or eating, and don't see yourself loathing any kind of food. The body needs food, but moderation is key.

Your subconscious mind will guide you to eat the foods in the right quantities if you visualize your body how you want it to look.

Exercise, dancing, being with friends, working at your job, being with your spouse, etc., are all good things to imagine.

Imagine yourself hearing people complimenting you about how good you look and admiring your slim body all the time.

Get as real as you can with the mental image.

Whenever you visualize weight loss, don't tell yourself, "well, it is all nonsense. I can't lose weight." By saying these words, you destroy all of your progress.

When thoughts of disbelief crawl into your mind, do not listen to them. Let only thoughts of your ideal body shape enter your mind.

The most important thing is to believe in yourself. Forget about your failed weight loss attempts and reject negative thinking, doubts, and disbelief.

Your disbelief and inner resistance will gradually fade away if you keep seeing your ideal figure in your mind.

Remember that results can take some time. Nothing happens overnight. You have to persist with the visualization day after day. In some cases, weight loss won't take very long, and in others, it will take more time.

If you want results, you need to persist in your efforts and not give up.

My own journey of leaving emotional eating and overeating behind has been made possible by the power of visualization.

I don't think the key lies in picturing our physical body but in envisioning the way we'll feel once we've conquered our challenges and obsessions with weight, food, the perfect body, that layer of fat in our stomach, or whatever it is that keeps you restricted and dieting.

The real change in my life started when I stopped looking at those unrealistic images and started picturing a future me who was free and happy and never had to diet.

You could just enjoy life, be confident, playful, relaxed, and just have fun. From sitting down to eat to playing, having fun, working, spending time with friends, exercising, and every time I saw myself, I focused (and still do to this day) on the part of myself that was totally free.

It's not about perfecting your body. It's about living a life that's free from food fears, it's about not overeating for self-soothing, and it's about feeling light.

The feeling of freedom and happiness that only comes from being at peace with yourself, imperfections and all.

Chapter 8: Meditation

Before starting with the concept of meditation, we would take a glance at what mindfulness is.

The tendency to rush through life without noticing much can be all too common.

Mindfulness is the act of being aware of your own thoughts and feelings, as well as the world around you. It's called mindfulness, and it can help us enjoy life and get to know ourselves better. You can make it happen in your own life if you want to.

You're mindful when you're paying attention to what's happening inside and outside of yourself.

People can become disconnected from the world around them. They can also lose touch with the way their bodies are feeling and end up living "in their heads" - lost in their thoughts without noticing how they influence their emotions and behaviors.

Mindfulness is all about paying attention to our body and what it's feeling. A simple thing like the feel of a banister when you walk upstairs can be a big part of mindfulness.

Mindfulness practice is also about being aware of your thoughts and feelings as they happen.

Being more present can help us understand ourselves and enjoy the world around us.

We start experiencing new things when we become more aware of the present moment.

Practicing mindfulness can also help us become more aware of how our thoughts and feelings flow and how we get entangled in those thoughts and feelings.

Slowly, we can train ourselves to understand that thoughts are simply "mental events" and that we don't have to be controlled by them.

Taking a step back and asking, "Are my thoughts really helping me solve this problem, or am I just getting caught up in them?" can be helpful when dealing with problems.

To practice mindfulness, you have to remind yourself to pay attention to your thoughts, feelings, body sensations, and everything around you.

Our daily lives are filled with sensations, whether it's the food we eat or the air passing by our bodies as we walk.

During a regular time, like a morning commute or lunchtime walk, try to pay attention to the sensations created by the world around you.

You'll also see the world in a whole new way if you try new things, like sitting in a different seat during meetings or going somewhere new for lunch.

Practicing mindfulness can be hard for some people because when they stop, all their thoughts and worries flood in.

Mindfulness isn't about getting rid of these thoughts but about seeing them as mental events that come and go. This can be hard at first, but with a little perseverance, you'll get there.

People find that doing gentle yoga or walking helps them cope with overthinking.

It can be helpful to silently name thoughts and feelings, like "Here's the thought that I might fail that exam" or *"Here's anxiety."*.

A mindful approach can be especially helpful if you're stuck reliving past problems or worrying about the future for several minutes.

Setting aside time for mindfulness practice can be helpful, along with practicing mindfulness every day.

Meditating with mindfulness involves sitting quietly and paying attention to thoughts, sounds, breathing sensations, or parts of your body, bringing your attention back whenever you start to drift.

Nowadays, meditation is one of the biggest things we're supposed to do. In addition to physical and mental health benefits, meditation and mindfulness are praised for their cognitive benefits too.

Both healthy people and sick people are supposed to benefit from meditation. It's said to calm you down mentally, physically, and cognitively.

Developing your breathing awareness can also be helped by yoga and tai-chi.

There's evidence that mindfulness can help with stress, anxiety, and depression. More research is needed to see if it helps with anything else.

There's no one-size-fits-all when it comes to mindfulness. Some people find that it helps, while others find that it makes them feel worse.

Now coming back to meditation. You might ask what meditation really is, or is meditation what you're looking for?

Before you think you know what meditation is, you should know what it's not. Meditation isn't zoning out or having earth-shattering experiences, or even controlling your mind.

Meditation is more about awareness, not zoning out. When you work on your mind, you'll feel more present, calm, attentive, and more empathic and patient.

There are a lot of things in life that are beyond our control, but we can have a lot more control over our actions and how we deal with the things we encounter.

In order to achieve this, we have to cultivate awareness of what the mind is doing and focus. And meditation is the best way to cultivate awareness.

We learn from Buddhist meditation that taking charge of our minds is the most crucial human endeavor. But we also learn that controlling your mind isn't what it's all about!

The key is connecting to our mind's natural qualities - spaciousness, goodness, creativity - so the light of our mind outshines the shadows of confusion and distress. A free mind finds its own peace.

"The way to control sheep or cows is to give them a spacious meadow,"

-Zen master Suzuki Roshi.

If we weren't for our minds, we'd be machines. Our knowledge, memories, joys, and sorrows; motor control, artistic skills, anger, love... everything!

But how much time do we devote to getting to know this mind? To train it? With meditation, we train our minds to be aware and relaxed instead of always focused on the external world as we do. And reveal its mind-boggling qualities!

Putting it another way, meditation is awareness. When we meditate, we devote a certain amount of time and effort to being as mindful as possible.

We choose an object to meditate on, like the breath. When we sit on a cushion or a chair, we stay upright and still, and we just pay attention to our breath.

As we breathe in, we're aware of it. When we breathe out, we're aware of it. Whenever we meditate, we find our minds don't stay put!

One minute we're focusing on the breath, the next moment, we're thinking about booking a flight to Paris or telling a colleague what we really think of her.

Getting to know the mind and learning to use its power starts with giving it space to express itself. Mind is creative and wants to be heard.

When we realize we've wandered from our breath, we gently but firmly invite the mind to come back. And then the mind wanders off.

And we bring it back again and again. It's a way to practice mindfulness, to meditate. As time goes by, we realize how peaceful and rich it is to be present, and pulling ourselves away becomes harder and harder.

You can watch videos where cows are let out for the first time in spring after spending winter in a barn.

Eventually, they settle down and ruminate contentedly, and the novelty wears off.

They frolic, kick, sniff, graze, and enjoy themselves immensely. We learn that happiness comes from contentment and presence in meditation.

Our happiness isn't based on external factors or material pursuits. Instead, it's based on how we learn to tap into the wealth of qualities already in us when we meditate.

Getting in touch with our most essential qualities, goodness and compassion, let us naturally express them in the world around us. That's what meditation does.

I've been interested in meditation for years. I meditated almost every day, using some of the popular guided meditations and mindfulness apps available.

After a while, my interest waned, and my practice stopped. Although I "felt" I had gained a few benefits, I wasn't really satisfied with the time commitment and the fact that I didn't see more profound results from my meditation practice.

There's a lot of confusion around meditation, so maybe I had wrong expectations, or maybe I wasn't meditating right. Still, I'm getting more confused about what meditation is and what types of meditation are out there.

Research on meditation also echoes this sentiment about how difficult it is to classify meditation.

There's still a lot of confusion about meditation since it's infused with local culture and religion and bantered around in the popular culture.

The word mindfulness is a similar problem. It has long left whatever meaning it used to hold historically and philosophically, and it now just means staying in the moment when washing the dishes or eating.

Meditation is difficult to define. Basically, I've realized the importance of distinguishing between different methods and techniques of meditating and their intended goals.

We're going to look at some other benefits of meditation too, but at its core, meditation was meant to help you think differently or shift your consciousness.

Meditating helped Buddha and others learn about themselves and the universe.

As more people find out about its health benefits, meditation is becoming more popular.

People use it to reduce stress and develop concentration. It can increase awareness about yourself and your surroundings.

As well as developing good habits and feelings, people use this practice for self-control, self-discipline, sleeping better, and even tolerating pain better.

CONCENTRATION MEDITATION

The purpose of concentration meditation is to focus on a single thing. This might be following your breath, repeating a single word, staring at a candle flame, listening to repetitive gongs, or counting beads on a mala.

For beginners, focusing the mind is tough, so they might only meditate for a few minutes and then work up to longer periods of time.

When you notice your mind wandering, simply refocus your awareness on the chosen object of attention.

Instead of following random thoughts, you let them go. Through this process, your concentration improves.

MINDFULNESS MEDITATION

By practicing mindfulness meditation, you acknowledge and observe wandering thoughts as they pass through your mind.

The goal isn't to judge or get involved with them but simply to be aware of what's happening right now.

During mindfulness meditation, you notice how your thoughts and feelings tend to move in a certain way.

Practicing will help you become more aware of your tendency to judge experiences quickly. With time, an inner balance will come.

A combination of concentration and mindfulness is taught in some schools of meditation. Many disciplines require stillness - to a greater or lesser extent.

OTHER MEDITATION TECHNIQUES

Among Buddhist monks, a daily meditation practice focuses on cultivating compassion, so there are lots of other meditation techniques.

The idea is to imagine negative events in a positive light and then transform them with compassion. You can also do moving meditation like tai chi, qigong, or walking meditation.

It makes me think of Buddhist monks mastering meditation on their way to enlightenment and wisdom when I think of mindfulness.

I think of the old monk meditating on life's meaning on top of a mountain. In its true form, meditation will facilitate this, as it's about focusing on one thought or idea and emptying our minds of extraneous noise, leading to heightened consciousness.

There's no need to be Zen masters in life. In reality, we all have aspects of life following us around. You don't have to be so focused on this very moment and action that everything else gets thrown out.

When we've got work, families, and stuff to do, we can't have some single-minded focus. I have to pay the mortgage, or I have to work on something at work that makes my mind go to work.

There are many benefits to mindfulness, and it doesn't mean that you have to sit in a lotus position for hours on end to practice it.

You can also carry mindfulness through your life and career by carrying yourself in your actions every day. In order to overcome any situation, you need to be aware of your thoughts, actions, and words.

You're your thoughts. Everything starts with them. If you think badly and make bad decisions throughout your career and life, it's only going to make things hard.

Relationships can get destroyed, or you can sabotage your career. What do you think of others? Do you see them as competitors or roadblocks to your success?

Are you looking at people as tools to get ahead? You may not think highly of some people, but do you see the goodness in them? Do you believe in the uniqueness and contribution of each individual?

Consider your upbringing, race, or gender when you take some time to empathize with them. Your thoughts determine who we are and how we act.

When you find yourself thinking negatively, force yourself to break this train of thought and consciously try to find something positive in the world.

Some people aren't likable or respectful, and they're responsible for their own choices, but don't think poisonous thoughts because they'll drip into your words and actions.

Look at everything in your career as an opportunity to grow and learn. Maybe the market isn't working, or maybe management isn't good, but ultimately you're responsible for how you think.

You can choose to be positive or negative, and your actions and success will change. Do you see something that needs improving? Are you working to fix it, or are you working to provide solutions?

Everything starts with your thoughts. Don't fall into negative thought patterns if you're mindful of this.

Life and work are full of words. Words can build relationships, and they can also destroy them. Are you critical of others when you speak with them? When you work, do you gossip, or do you actively attack others?

It's a cliché, but it's also true that if you have nothing positive to say, you might want to think twice about saying it.

Is it likely that people will want to communicate with you if you are seen as someone who is always complaining about things or spewing negative things about people?

It's true that there are people who engage in devious activities, and things won't always be perfect, but if you're contributing to a conversation that doesn't have a positive tone, you might ask others to stop or move away.

The more positive the words you say, the more genuine the relationship will be.

You'll have more opportunities down the road if you communicate well with your coworkers, management, and customers.

You can cultivate respect from others, create stronger relationships, and get more career opportunities through mindful thinking, actions, and words.

There's no big shift. You just need to pay more attention. For people who think ill of others all the time or default to negative tendencies, it's more difficult.

A few moments of calming thoughts or a quick pause can cure negativity quickly and easily. It doesn't require learning meditation techniques, changing your religion, or moving to another area to be mindful.

After meditation comes the part where most meditators find ways to delve themselves into deep meditation.

If you think you're not making progress in deep meditation, you might be tempted to switch techniques. But this won't solve the problem. It takes patience, time, and training to master any kind of meditation.

We explore the connection between body and mind through mindfulness, which is a key part of any meditation practice.

Our aim is to stay aware of what we're doing without getting swept away by thoughts and feelings, like the pleasurable feelings you get with deep meditation.

With everything going so fast in our busy world, we often feel like time is moving so fast.

Taking time to practice deep meditation can help us cope with today's frenzied pace. These feelings are completely normal, but they lead to anxiety and stress.

Most people might be unaware of the fact that meditation can actually help someone in their weight loss journey.

If you're eating well and managing your weight and your health, it's important to acknowledge the mind-body connection.

If you feel weighed down by your hectic, jam-packed life, don't worry. You're not alone if you feel this way.

The good news is that there are steps you can take that might be able to help you lose or manage weight, and meditation is one of them.

Meditating, mindful eating, and intuitive eating are some of the things we can learn or relearn to have a healthy relationship with food, as well as to get rid of any negative feelings we may have.

It's okay to lose weight if you cultivate this renewed relationship, but don't make losing weight the main goal. That could make it hard for us to really eat intuitively or mindfully.

Rather than stressing about work or family issues and feeling overwhelmed, enjoy food - eat because you're hungry, not because you're overwhelmed. You'll learn how to love your body through this practice.

Emotional eating or stress eating happens when people eat and overeat based on their emotions instead of responding to their hunger cues.

Often, when we're feeling strong, our feelings of fullness and satiation can outweigh our physical feelings, so we overeat.

People use food as a coping mechanism, dulling out strong emotions for a while. Stress can cause overeating, which in turn can cause guilt or shame, which leads to feeling - and not being able to handle - negative emotions or stress.

If you're having trouble with food or eating experiences, you can use mindful eating.

You have to be present and pay attention to how the food tastes, smells and feels — it's about being present.

To slow down and listen to our internal cues of true hunger versus cues of satiation, mindful eating incorporates intuitive eating. This helps us reduce emotional eating or binge eating.

It's true that mindful eating can lead to weight loss, but weight loss shouldn't be the goal. If we're eating for a specific physical outcome, we've already abandoned mindful eating.

It's not uncommon for people to think about spinning classes or salads instead of burgers when it comes to losing weight.

It's counterintuitive to think about sitting in one place and focusing on your thoughts, and doing a meditation for weight loss. But those kinds of perceptions are just a part of the truth.

Getting in shape isn't just about physical stuff, and it's not just black and white.

It's important to acknowledge that we're emotional beings when we're trying to develop a healthy relationship with food, lose body fat, or keep our weight at a healthy weight.

We have a group of information communicators called neurotransmitters between our brain's 100 billion neurons.

Our pick-me-up neurotransmitters are serotonin and norepinephrine, which help us feel good when we're down.

The names sound familiar because antidepressants often target one or both of these chemicals (and not as well as they used to).

It's estimated that as many as 25 percent of people taking antidepressants gain weight. And sometimes a lot of weight, up to 100 pounds.

It's clear that finding a NATURAL way to boost these two pleasure chemicals has no side effects, despite the fact that it can be caused by carb cravings or slowed metabolism.

Meditation uncaps our happy juice fire hydrant naturally.

Researchers have found that ancient mind practices boost serotonin and norepinephrine to levels that beat depression right in the face.

Our brains are naturally flooded with these two pleasure chemicals, so we don't need food to feel good all the time.

Meditation is something anyone can do. No special equipment is needed, and there aren't expensive classes to attend. For most people, finding the time is the hardest part. Try starting out with 10 minutes a day or even every other day.

Try to schedule these 10 minutes around your children's waking time or after they go to bed to minimize distractions. You can even do it in the shower if you don't have a quiet place.

Make yourself comfortable in a quiet place. You can lie down or sit however feels good to you.

Take a moment to focus on your breath, watching your chest and stomach rise and fall.

Feel the air moving in and out of your mouth or nose. Listen to the sounds the air makes. Do this for a minute or two until you feel relaxed.

Here's what you need to do, with or without your eyes open:

Breathe in deeply and hold it for a minute.

Take a deep breath and exhale slowly.

Let your body breathe.

Pay attention to your breath as it enters your nose, lifts your chest, or moves your belly, but don't change it.

Spend five to ten minutes just focusing on your breath.

There will be times when your mind wanders, which is totally normal. Just acknowledge it and return your attention to your breathing.

Consider how easy it was to let your mind wander as you wrap up. Then, acknowledge how easy it was to get back on track.

Remember that when you start doing it, it might feel hard and uncomfortable at first. But with regular practice, it'll get easier and feel more natural.

Mindful eating is about paying attention to the taste and texture of your meals by chewing slowly and thinking about what you taste in each bite while you eat without distractions.

When you're trying to lose weight, you should add meditation to your diet and exercise plan. It's possible to lose weight and stay fit if you eat mindfully and meditate. When you do it right, you won't feel ashamed, judged, or harsh.

Chapter 9: Source Energy

Everyone in the spiritual world believes humans have a connection to source energy, whether it's psychic, intuitive, healer, channeler, or anything else.

It might be higher intelligence, God, universal law, or something else. It doesn't have a label. We just call it 'source energy'.

We can never be separated from source energy. We can't ever be cut off from it, no matter how much we feel disconnected from it.

As soon as we are conceived, we stretch that connection so we can live our human adventure. As soon as we die, we rejoin it fully, joining it all together.

That doesn't mean we're ever not part of the whole, but sometimes it feels like that.

It makes us feel secure knowing we're never alone because we can always tap into the infinite from where we came. A connection to the source gives us faith and helps us cope with life's demands.

When we are children, we experience boundless curiosity, energy, and a feeling of connection to all that is.

We incline to let nature have its way with us since we are animals infused with spirit before becoming conscious humans.

Our civilization's dualistic thinking would have kept us from losing our connection to body, mind, and spirit, along with our connection to the universe through our hearts.

It's a journey that everyone needs to take for themselves to rediscover this kind of connection in this era of high-speed, high-tech changes.

Ever felt energized by an inspiring movie, transformed by a great symphony, or held spellbound by a life-affirming book?

Was it a moment when you walked away feeling good, only to say to a friend, "That made life seem logical.".

I wish life were more like that! But maybe life can be more like that, with a greater sense of clarity. If life seems like a puzzle, you might just be missing parts!

As wonderful and healing as it is to foster greater connections with humans and with the earth, I have been taking it a step further in recent years.

Through a kind of broadband connection of the spirit, I have been able to reach out to what I have gradually come to know as "The Source" to address any issue.

In the end, it is the place where all creative ideas and creative energies originate from. The Source is not a physical place, but a place within ourselves, one we can access through consciousness.

Known also as source energy, this life force flows through and connects all things. The manifestations of this life energy are everywhere.

When we become more attuned to and work with this gold mine of consciousness, we can make our lives more miraculous than anything we can imagine.

I do what is called focalizing, a method of discovering and working with source energy. Meditation, trauma resolution, and creative pursuits are some of the pathways to this.

With both a healing and a creative component, focalizing can encourage a continuous flow of energy through us and allow this energy to express itself more clearly.

It is an enlivening current we can feel in our bones, whether we call it spirit, God, a higher power, or the universe, but we can call it spirit, God, a higher power, or the universe.

Some may experience it as a vibration, some as stillness, others as a presence. Regardless of how you describe it, the source energy is a universal force found in all living things.

Plants align themselves towards the sun due to their universal intelligence, which is why it is full of universal intelligence.

Our bodies also speak to us when we listen to them, and we can use them to make better decisions.

Having conditioned thinking can make it difficult for us to shift our perceptions and heal our lives, since it refers back to past experiences and exposures. It regurgitates old information and story lines that have been passed down from generation to generation.

With both healing and creativity, focalizing can help us express our energy in a more clear way.

Intricacy is not well tolerated by the conditioned mind and may make it difficult for the mind to deal with love, joy, and other more complex and subtle aspects of life.

When we are not equipped with new tools and a fresh way to see, our minds can hold us back and prevent us from making the best decisions we can.

The heart's intelligence, on the other hand, thrives on nuance and complexity and on the connection to deep ancestral roots.

Through felt sensations of our bodies and sensory perceptions, it guides our next steps on the path to becoming a fully realized person.

As our hearts guide us through a natural, fulfilling process of connection, we respectfully set aside our minds and let our hearts guide us through one thing.

We might become aware of the role the body plays in shaping our mind and our moment-to-moment experience as we host source energy. By doing so, we may be able to shift from experiencing with our senses to experiencing with awareness.

By consciously directing our minds to be aware, we may be able to access subtle options that we cannot access simply by thinking.

In order to host this energy, we can take a deep breath. We can also practice a body drop. During a body drop, awareness is focused on deeply relaxing the body while remaining connected to it. This is referred to as "striving only to be."

When we take a moment to breathe, we gain flexibility, allowing our mind to switch between its outwardly focused mind and its subtler inner mind, which uses feelings.

As we develop this skill, we may be able to employ both levels of awareness fluidly, enhancing our sense of inner knowing and developing a fluid sense of awareness.

In this way, the imagined division between body, mind, and nature can be unified, and source energy can be energized to provide guidance.

Our experience of time collapses in this embodied state, allowing us to connect with imagery and perceptions that are often deeply informative and enlightening. With this focalizing, we can rediscover the lost connections we see in children's and wild animals' eyes.

Getting contentment and happiness does not require wagging a magic wand or snapping our fingers.

The choices are based on an acceptance of what is exactly as it is and respect for present realities because reality is constantly changing.

Don't disconnect from reality. Accept things as they are and let source energy transform them as it sees fit.

We can often maintain, host, and rely on the established connection to source energy in order to keep our loving relationship with spirit vibrant and alive. This can be accomplished with gratitude.

The only way to un-separate ourselves from the source of energy if we ever feel we lack gratitude for being alive is to un-separate ourselves from it.

When we are connected to the wellspring of spiritual creativity, we cannot help but feel joyful, playful, and grateful.

We can become the change we wish to see in the world by releasing our preconceived concepts about who we are and becoming one with the source of energy.

External sources of higher power can be described as God, goddess, god, the universe, etc. Each source of higher power resonates differently with each person.

As one wades gradually into the world of healing practices, it's important to keep this in mind. No two people, their experiences, or beliefs are the same.

Healers with intuitive guidance listen deeply to the guidance they receive from these external sources about what blockages need to be removed, whether mentally, emotionally, physically, or spiritually.

"There's a direct correlation between positive energy and positive results."

-Joe Regan

Our personal development really comes down to one thing and one thing only: aligning ourselves with our source of energy. When we feel connected to our source energy, we feel like we're flying.

This is the energy that heals the body and the emotions. It is the energy that revitalizes the body. It is the energy that renews the soul. It is the energy that gives us life.

Inspiration and motivation come directly from it. You will be driven to dream bigger and accomplish your goals through it. It's what will make your life the best it can be.

If you always feel connected to the source, never feeling disconnected, stressed, or uncertain, then this post is for you. If you feel confused, stressed, or uncertain, then please keep reading.

The more you know that source is always with you - because it is you and you are it - the better you'll feel. Knowing divine guidance is among you - continually - is incredibly empowering.

Why do you think we're connected to Source?

This spark, or divine essence, is what you tap into when you work with your intuition, when you seek inner wisdom, or when you have thought of inspiration.

Regardless of what spiritual development work you do, I believe that you're developing a connection with 'source.'

A big part of why you are here is not only to experience being a real human being but also to remember that you are the source of everything.

If you want to start connecting with yourself, make a habit of checking in with your body every day. Our body tends to speak more quietly than our Ego mind does.

To start with, let's get clear on what the Ego mind is and does. Often, when we talk about our Ego, we think of it as something bad, like arrogance or pride.

Ultimately, the Ego-mind is our survival mechanism; it's part of what keeps us alive, and it's connected to our fight-or-flight response.

The way we're living our lives under constant stress has caused us to be stressed out, and our ego-minds have become overworked, so we're always in a fight-or-flight state.

We haven't necessarily had bad Ego-minds, but we have learned to act on the limited information they provide after receiving it first.

We need to re-program this pattern, so the Ego-mind knows it's OK to step out of survival mode and rest.

As we practice affirmations regularly, we provide reassurance, acceptance, appreciation, and compassion to the Ego-mind so it can be re-taught.

The Ego-mind might make it hard for some people to practice compassion when they realize that it's a part of themselves.

Trying to practice compassion for our parts, including the Ego-mind, can be easier if you look at them from a third-party perspective.

Acceptance is part of our survival needs, so shame and judgment have to go. This can trigger an egoic survival response. We can only teach the Ego-mind safety and security if we reassure, accept, and compassionately treat it.

Getting in touch with your body by doing daily body check-ins can help you to determine your personal energy baseline and help you become more aware of when something might need attention or be out of balance.

It's gonna help you use your discernment better if you know how energies outside of yourself are affecting you, if you know what it feels like being in your body, recognizing the energies coursing through your veins.

The more you pay attention to this, the more you'll notice the connection we all have with everything and everyone.

Every day, we strive for new experiences. We all think we're chasing our dreams and desires, but they're nothing but experiences of life.

With the realization of the source, your life transcends forever. You see the same world with a different perception. Each experience of life fades away in time, but the experience of the source stays forever.

Your entire view of life changes with your perception. The first and last goal of life should be to connect with the source. We all have different goals, but we have never looked for them.

"Source Energy is ALWAYS flowing through you!"

It's important to do certain things that remind you of your source. These things will help you to feel connected. When you allow the flow to run its course completely, the joy will be yours.

Be still. Breathe steadily and relax. Feel source energy fill your body and aura. You don't have to meditate or visualize. Just be still. You don't have to concentrate.

Take a walk or sit in the fresh air. Focus on breathing. Feel the source energy envelope you and revitalize you. Go to the beach, a lake, the mountains, the desert, fields - anywhere peaceful where the air is fresh.

You are with people you love. As you are with them, enjoying their company, laughing, talking, crying, loving, sympathizing, or simply enjoying their presence, let yourself feel the comfort as energy. It's your source, wrapping you in love.

Feel the excitement as you do what you love. Appreciate different colors, sounds, words, smells, and whatever you're doing. Being creative, inspired, and enthusiastic is a powerful feeling.

It's like we're constantly being told to 'reach for our full potential,' like we're less than until we get there. We can fulfill our potential in any area of our lives, whether it's in our careers or spiritually.

You don't need to become a CEO or a Zen master. You're already perfect right where you are.

Allowing is all you need to do. You can't do anything, take no courses, or get any qualifications. You just have to allow it.

In letting go, you let go of anxiety and worries because you know it's all going to be alright. You know everything's going to be okay, and it's okay not to have to control every detail or manipulate the outcome. Rather than fighting against the forces of the universe, it's about surrendering to them.

By allowing, you let yourself be inspired, allow yourself to be guided by the flow, and simply do what needs to be done at the moment.

One thing at a time. Allowing yourself to let go of the shoulds, musts, and guilts that weigh you down.

Allowing constantly will become second nature, and you will be able to recognize when you are being overwhelmed by stressful thoughts and tap into your inner serenity instantly.

An energy system is commonly found in open cultures, with energy points located throughout the body. If magic is internal to the body, then it comes from the mind or the body.

An individual's veins or brain can become suffused with it, depending on how much is used. Another possibility is that it is merely a mental function, like reading or doing calculations, without any tangible existence.

So long as the magic user isn't dependent on outer means, magic's source is internal, even if it can be enhanced by them.

Among the external sources are The Spirit of the World, a God, a magical artifact, and similar entities.

It is necessary to draw from that source before using magic in this case. According to the nature of the source, it can be achieved either through specific actions, such as prayer or ritual, or via a conduit, such as an object or a person.

Our understanding of energy can be simplified if we get quiet and feel into ourselves or our surroundings. If we get quiet and feel into ourselves or our surroundings, we can understand energy better.

Whenever we feel present, our energy is grounded; if we feel attraction or repulsion, our energy may be charged; when we laugh or cry, our energy may be discharged.

We can lose our energy if we're in certain situations or with certain people. Alternatively, if we don't feel like we're enough, we might cling to someone else's fuel.

Energy is everything. When we want to create separation, we bind our energy, and when we want to get close, we let our energy flow freely.

Energy can't be created or destroyed - but it can be altered. That's the first thing we learn in school. Speeding up or slowing down energy is possible.

Depending on whether the energy is held or bound in a closed system or if it flows openly, it can exist in either.

System fragmentation can happen when there's too much-uncontained energy. System collapse can happen when the energy is depleted.

It's a neutral force, even though it has a lot of power. Consciousness is what drives its movement.

As we think about energy and consciousness in terms of the human experience, it may make sense to observe that the more conscious we are, the more we create, connect, and evolve.

It's more common for our energy to be used towards separation, stagnation, or even destruction, the less conscious we are.

You can gain strength in deep transition by focusing on two main energy channels. The first one is grounding to the center of Mother Earth. Mother Earth is our mother, and our bodies come from the matter that makes up the Earth.

Mater means "mother." She's the one who gives us everything we need. She's got the air we breathe, the water we drink, the food we eat, and shelter for us.

It's like she's supporting us every step of the way. There's something alive about Mother Earth, and she's ascended into a higher world.

We're all on this ride together!Connecting with the Earth empowers your creativity, supports your health, and energizes your being. She's got a great energy channel that you should connect to daily.

Your energy should be directed into your feet and tailbone, then sending it deep into the earth, past the roots of the trees, the layers of soil, the bedrock, the underground streams and caverns, and into the heart of your Mother.

As you breathe in, visualize her nourishment spiraling up like a river into your feet and legs, tailbone, and perineum. As you breathe out, visualize your own nourishment spiraling up into her.

Continually breathe in her energy up and exhale your nervous tension into her, which she will transmute. Do this exercise for 5-10 minutes until you can feel her energy filling your body, feeling completely connected.

Whenever you are flooded with thoughts, it will calm you down, and you will feel grounded and supported. You will feel like you are filling up.

By saying the words out loud, you are creating a reality by emulating sound. Each statement you make out loud is transformed into a reality by the sound you produce.

The words you speak create your reality. You speak all your words into existence.

In order to connect with the spiritual sun, which is the heart of the universe, you must first connect with the spiritual sun, which is the heart of Universe.

Your energy should be sent up into the Universe from your Crown chakra on top of your head, through the atmosphere of Earth, into space, through the stars and galaxies, until you feel connected to the Universe's core.

By stating your intention, "I am connecting with the heart of the Universe." Once you feel you have reached that place, say out loud, "I AM one with the heart of the Universe." You will feel a higher frequency entering your energy field and being.

As you breathe deeply here, connect the earth's energy and the Universal energy, where they will intertwine. You will feel lighthearted as a result.

A tube of light or energy spiral feeds your body and energy field with the vital energy needed to evolve. This channel supplies your body and energy field with the vital energy it needs to evolve.

Grounding exercises work on your root chakra when you feel anxious or fearful, and Universal energy exercises work on your crown chakra when you feel depressed.

Performing this exercise for 10-15 minutes each day will make a big difference! As you practice, you will experience greater well-being, and your spirals will become larger.

It takes so much to stay balanced in these times. Just keeping a positive mental attitude can sometimes be challenging.

Spend time with those you love, and take excellent care of yourself. There is no doubt that you will succeed.

These intense times make it important for us to take care of ourselves. Through the light codes streaming from the Spiritual

Sun, our physical bodies are being upgraded, and our DNA is being upgraded, too.

As we ascend, our bodies are going through a transformation, and it's going to make us tired, drained, and irritable. We're also clearing out karma and old energy.

We let go of so much and face loss, and there's the deep pain that goes with it. It's okay to be sensitive and grieving as we let go of so much.

Be kind, patient, and loving to yourself on this journey. Love all sides of yourself, especially the part where you're insecure, lonely, and afraid.

If you let go of control, you'll feel in control. It will give you calm, energy, and inspiration.

You'll know it's natural to have changeable moods, and you won't beat yourself up when you're feeling low for a bit.

You know it will soon pass, and you'll be back on track. You look for things to appreciate because you know appreciation means love.

You'll change your life. You'll always have faith in your source. People will be drawn to you. When they're with alignment

They'll leave you happier than they were when they arrived. You're able to tune in to your inner guidance whenever you want to. It helps you get closer to the Divine and trust your source more.

Our lives aren't aligned very often...we work for a job that stifles our values, stay in relationships that smother our true selves and make choices about our time that ignore who we are and what we care about.

Having this kind of existence can make us feel cynical, hopeless, angry, self-loathing, and unsatisfied with our lives in general.

In essence, alignment is the expression of what it feels and looks like to be connected with yourself and live in harmony with your deepest truths. It's also what brings us the most happiness and peace of mind.

We're not living an authentic life if we're not in alignment with ourselves because we're not true or in agreement with ourselves.

It's inevitable that when we try to pretend to be someone else, or if we try to fulfill someone else's wants, wants, and expectations, we'll create friction.

There's a lot of friction, and it leaves us feeling exhausted and depleted. Eventually, this leads to feelings of overwhelm, stress, and anxiety, which may manifest physically or emotionally.

It's important to stay true to yourself, to live according to your values, and to keep your mind and soul aligned.

The more aligned we are, the easier it becomes to flow with life. For example, let's say you get a lot of pressure from your family to get a good degree, so you study medicine, but you soon realize that you don't like those classes.

But you have an elective in the art that you love and always look forward to.

Even though you're sure you'd like art classes more than science courses, you still have a voice inside your head telling you that business courses will help you get ahead in life and pay the bills.

Last but not least, life isn't static. We cancel plans, we break up with people, our bodies change, and we find new passions.

Say you've been running for most of your life, but now you're in your 50s, and your body can't handle that level of exercise.

You can keep pushing your body to the limit or find something new that's equally satisfying. Changing plans makes us feel bad. Rather than seeing it as a problem, I challenge you to look at it as an opportunity.

When we let go of the things we're not in control of, doors open that we never dreamed were there.

Of course, things won't always work out the way we expect, but what if we asked, "What are the new adventures I'm going to have now that I'm on a different path?"?"

Our alignment begins and ends with listening to our hearts and bodies. When we look inward, we can gain so much insight into who we are and what doesn't fulfill us.

Once we've found that level of alignment with ourselves, we can steer our energy toward the things that bring us happiness and peace. When we do that, the world becomes better and happier.

Chapter 10: Journaling

Keeping a journal or diary can lead to many different benefits for you, but understanding what journaling is and what its benefits are, can often be confusing.

This chapter is intended to help you get a better understanding of journaling.

When you journal, you write down your deepest thoughts and feelings, then put them on paper to express yourself.

In order to handle life's difficulties and uncertainties, journaling builds strong "emotional muscles" for mental, emotional, and spiritual health.

Journaling helps you discover your sense of purpose and meaning in life, as well as your relationship with a higher power, by identifying your negative thoughts and beliefs and replacing them with positive, healing ones.

While journaling has been around for thousands of years, it's just coming into its own right now.

Even though it's getting more popular lately, it's not just a new-age self-help trend. If you practice it consistently, you'll have better mental, emotional, and physical health.

Sometimes journaling is restorative. Sometimes it helps us to feel grateful for those around us. Sometimes it helps us capture those thoughts that help us feel gratitude for those around us.

It encourages you to dig deep into an emotional exploration, channeling feelings into a way to express yourself that inspires growth and discovery.

No matter how old you are or how busy you are, keeping a journal for just a few minutes during the day can be a great thing.

Writing down your thoughts and feelings is a great way to deal with everyday life.

It's a deeply personal experience that can take many forms, but there's no right or wrong way to journal.

You can journal one day and write a diary entry like you used to when you were a teenager. The next day you could write down things you like or things you want to accomplish in your life.

You can gain meaningful insights into yourself, grow and become more self-aware when you journal, especially when you're feeling anxious or sad.

Those are the reasons journaling is great for self-improvement.

As part of the self-care movement, journaling has been on top of meditation and teenage girls for a long time. Science has proved that meditation is basically a panacea for modern life.

You'll get better sleep, a stronger immune system, more self-confidence, and a higher I.Q., plus it boosts your mindfulness, memory, and communication skills. But research has also shown that writing in a journal can boost your sleep and your self-confidence.

There's something calming about writing down your thoughts at the end of the day, even if they weren't particularly positive.

Journaling for mental health has been shown to be beneficial because you can dump negative thoughts from your mind and reinforce positive ones.

Most people don't really know themselves and who they are. The benefits of keeping a journal are that you'll start to recognize patterns and triggers, and then you can learn how to deal with them.

It doesn't matter how old you are or how experienced you are, there's always room for improvement. Keeping a journal doesn't have to be a long-term process – it can be a way to track your progress during any given period, like during a new job trial period or counseling.

Many people have reported that keeping a journal helps to reduce anxiety and depression, though not all people do.

The very best part will be that it will help you develop a tool that you can take to your doctor or therapist. It will give them a better understanding of you, and you'll both be able to use it.

It's really useful to follow patterns and trends about yourself, not just to get to know yourself better and to identify things you should avoid and encourage, but also to learn about yourself.

Find out what you did differently or what happened differently if you're happier during particular weeks or days.

The most common question asked is, "What should I write about?"

When you start writing a journal, this is usually the first question you'll ask yourself too. However, in some ways, it's the most misguided — one lesson I've learned from journaling is that a mind is a weird place, and you don't know what you're looking for until you start knocking around in it.

Otherwise, you can't figure out what you should write about unless you write in your journal.

Whenever we sit down with a blank page, it can be frustrating and ineffective to figure out where to start. If we don't know if we're doing it right, we'll feel silly or embarrassed, and at worst, we might feel like our time is a waste.

Journaling allows us to explore our emotions and even ask ourselves these questions. For example, you can write about how silly you feel or why writing feels hard sometimes. When we have the space to vent or express our true feelings without judgment, it's like lifting a weight.

The best place to start is by asking questions, especially when you sit down and your mind instantly wanders to 'what on earth should I write about?'.

You can start beating that internal editor in your head by setting a timer before you write. Even if you just write, 'I don't know what to write anymore.'

Writing in this way will help you beat it. You won't have to rewrite, fix spelling mistakes, or criticize what you've written since you'll not be able to rewrite.

Making journal entries a daily habit rather than just an occasional hobby is the key to reaping all of the benefits of journaling.

When you write every day, you can gain insights, make breakthroughs, and work through difficult situations and emotions.

Keeping a journal is also a great mindfulness practice because it helps you stay present without worrying about the past or future. Being present without worrying about the past or future feels very calming and relaxing.

A daily journal can help you unload heavy feelings of stress by calming you down. A 20-minute journaling routine before bed can help you feel better.

It's a way to express yourself without judgment or rules, a place where positive and negative experiences can be channeled into something that makes you feel connected.

You don't need a degree in linguistics to keep a journal. Especially since journals are meant to be genuine and boundless expressions of your emotions.

Keeping a journal stimulates creativity and promotes well-being. It helps you develop strong writing habits, which translate into other skills like solving problems.

You'll be able to process information to clear your mind. This will improve your learning skills, contribute to your creativity, and help you:

- Make your creativity work for you
- Boost your productivity and focus
- You'll be able to manifest your goals faster
- Let your emotions and thoughts out

When you keep a consistent record of your life, you can monitor your patterns and behaviors over time. This history can show your growth and help you remember important things.

It's long been recognized that journaling can reduce stress, help with depression and anxiety, organize your life, focus your mind, and help you meditate. It can also be a great tool for opening up and letting go.

If you keep a journal, you can do it anytime, anywhere, and without having to dedicate much time, skill, or resources. Journaling is a lot more than just writing down what you think.

You can improve your mental health and get your life back on track by journaling every day, whether you're struggling with relationships, future goals, staying organized, or even in how you communicate with someone in your life, be it your partner, your kids, your coworkers, friends, your parents, or anything else.

When you express yourself creatively, like by writing in a journal, you relieve stress and focus on the things in your life that don't serve you.

Journals are great for establishing or practicing healthy habits, setting goals, managing mental health, and focusing on oneself.

Start a journal immediately if you've never written one. It can seem intimidating if you haven't journaled regularly in the past. However, writing a journal entry isn't as hard as you think it is.

Keep in mind that journaling is just a tool for processing your thoughts, bringing clarity to your emotions, and monitoring your thought patterns.

Anxiety is your body's natural response to stressful events. You don't have to worry or feel anxious all the time. But if it stops you from living your life, you may need to change.

When you think too much and talk too pessimistically, you can develop anxiety disorders or depression. Maybe you've tried all kinds of things to help with anxiety, but nothing works.

It's no secret that journaling is an effective coping strategy.

Writing down your worries can provide instant relief from anxiety. It allows you to face your fears and even embrace them. It makes you more vulnerable, so stress is reduced.

It's backed up by research, too. Positive affect journaling (PAJ) has been found to help with anxiety and depression. By writing down thoughts and feelings, people learn more about themselves and figure out what needs to get better.

People can talk about their thoughts and feelings, and it helps them identify them. Studies even recommend that PAJ should be included in routine anxiety treatment.

In a journal, you can write down everything that's stressing you without worrying about burdening those close to you. This is a healthy way to get your mind off your shoulders.

Try keeping a journal when you're having trouble making a decision, organizing a big project, feeling stressed, anxious, confused, or whatever.

The benefits of journaling go beyond just intellectual, organizational, and psychological benefits. Some studies show that it can also improve your physical health. And you don't have to be a good writer for any of these advantages.

In the last 20 years, artists, writers, psychotherapists, and even little girls who receive locked pink diaries have realized how important journal writing is. But did you know that scientists like Marie Curie and Albert Einstein kept journals too?

It's all about taking time to externalize your thoughts and feelings without fear of judgment from yourself or anyone else.

Journaling isn't about writing down your thoughts in an object or format — let alone if it'd pass muster with your high school English teacher — but about taking time to externalize what's on your mind.

Journals are great for problem-solving, expressing hidden or unacceptable feelings, and keeping track of creative ideas you might use for work or school. However, can keeping one improve your physical health?

There's evidence that writing can boost your immune system by reducing stress.

When you're feeling stressed, upset, or angry, it's easy to ignore it by scrolling on social media or binge-watching your favorite show. Let's face it, numbing your feelings is nothing new.

If you hide your feelings, they eventually have power, and you get chronic stress because of it. The more you bury them, the more powerful they become. Long-term stress can lead to heart problems and lowered immunity. Journaling can help with that.

Taking a few minutes to acknowledge and accept your emotions will allow you to release them and move forward in a healthier way. That sounds like mindfulness meditation, but it's different.

In spring, when the first blooms appear, bathing suit season is just around the corner. It's impossible to avoid exercising and eating well, but long-term weight loss starts in mind.

A healthy attitude can help you think and believe in healthy practices, experts say. Many people think about their activities and routines when trying to lose weight and get healthy, like what they eat and how they move, when it comes to losing weight and becoming healthier. We've got to change our attitudes and beliefs in addition to our physical activity in order to lose weight.

Journaling your food might seem like just another thing on your to-do list, but the time you invest could change everything.

You don't need to be a nerd to keep a food journal. You can record your meals in a notebook or a piece of paper throughout the day, or you can use a website or an app.

Losing weight means reducing mental fat, which will lower your waistline fat. To do that, you need to look at the patterns and habits that are holding you back.

Everybody has their own set of reasons. Most people manage to improve their lifestyles and nutrition until something goes wrong — whether it's work pressure, family problems, or something else. You have to break the pattern to succeed, whatever your issue is.

You'll be more successful at keeping a food journal if you keep track of your meals, snacks, and beverages consistently.

Almost everyone underestimates how much food they really eat. Break out those measuring cups and measuring spoons and learn how to serve yourself the right portions by using them (they can do more than just help you bake).

It won't take you long to figure out what portion sizes to eat when you go out for dinner away from home after using these items at home for several weeks.

It helps you notice behaviors that influence your eating habits so that you can change them through cognitive behavioral change.

Food journaling helps you recognize behavioral patterns. What percentage of calories do you consume after dinner? How many calories are in your lunch meal? Are you snacking too much during the day? Do you notice that you're consuming too many calories from sugary drinks? Are you overeating after a stressful day?

When you write it down and assess your food log, you often don't realize these behaviors are barriers to weight loss.

The more you write down your food intake, the more accountable you'll become to yourself, which motivates you to stick to it.

If a dietitian or other health professional analyzes your food journal and gives you detailed, specific advice, and gives you encouragement along the way, you're also responsible to them.

You can also see if you're eating a well-balanced diet by keeping a food journal. If you aren't, you'll soon figure out if there's any room for improvement in your diet.

You might think you're getting a lot of fruit and vegetables in your diet. A food journal will tell you whether you're really getting enough fruit and veggies.

When you're able to see at a glance what you've eaten that day, even a minor deficiency can become more obvious.

It's also possible to see if certain foods give you unpleasant aftereffects. For example, you may notice that you get gas or bloating pretty often when you eat a certain food but not with others.

This might be a sign that your body can't tolerate it very well, so you can decide whether to cut it out of your diet.

You probably knew you were getting these symptoms but didn't associate them with something you ate before you started keeping a food journal.

A food journal can help you lose weight and keep it off, according to studies. One study found that people who kept a food diary for six days a week lost twice as much weight as those who didn't do it or did it just one day a week.

In a food journal, you might see you're snacking a lot more than you're aware of, and if you also keep track of what you're doing at the time, you'll see that it's not really because you're hungry but because you're mindless.

If you're watching TV while you're eating, you might not be really appreciating what you're eating. You might not realize you've eaten a lot more than you thought.

The app can also help you figure out when you eat. For example, maybe you eat nothing during the day, and then you eat crazy things in the evenings. You can keep your appetite under control by being aware of this and spacing out your eating.

One of the best things you can do for yourself is to write a journal. Getting rid of layers of emotional gunk that's clogging up your body, mind, and spirit will keep your energy and emotions in low vibration.

If you're in a low vibrational state, you can't manifest what you want. By journaling regularly, you can release all those pent-up emotions and raise your vibration.

In other words, your life is created by how you think and act, according to the saying, *where your focus goes, your energy flows*.

It's crucial to practice mindfulness and choose your thoughts and intentions with self-awareness since the universe brings you what you focus on.

Getting high vibration means, basically, improving your mood. Getting out of your negative state and moving to something that feels good is what you can do through journaling your feelings.

Exchanging your thoughts from weakening worry to empowering gratitude. Experiencing love and kindness rather than anger or judgment. When you feel good, you radiate goodness. This world needs a lot of goodness right now!

According to metaphysics and science, humans have four energy levels: physical, mental, emotional, and spiritual.

Each of these levels vibrates at a specific frequency, and when they are combined, they create your overall state of being.

You're vibrating at a high frequency if you wake up every morning with a positive attitude, joy, motivation, and a sense of mission.

Alternatively, if you feel bored, demotivated, and melancholic, you're vibrating at a low frequency.

Keeping a high vibration will make you more productive and creative since a high vibration will make you feel light and energized, and at this point, I believe that journaling can help a lot to keep your vibrations high.

It's common for us to form habits that give us temporary gratification and relief when stressed out, so when stressed out, we self-medicate by acting destructively.

If you're overworking and not having a balanced lifestyle, then you might indulge in sugary food, drink alcohol, binge-watch TV, or do whatever you want.

This kind of behavior can't last long, and it keeps us feeling low, trapping us in this unhealthy cycle, and lowering our vibration.

Whenever we lower our vibration, we feel dark and heavy and like there's an empty void inside, and even if we have everything together in our lives, we can't fill it up.

A thought is a subtle form of energy in our brain that vibrates at a certain frequency. As you focus on a thought, it becomes stronger and stronger until it manifests into your reality.

Our emotions are energy in motion, and our thoughts affect our emotions and actions. If you think and write pessimistic or fearful thoughts regularly, you may find yourself drawn to situations that agree with them.

Human beings vibrate at a certain frequency, so we attract reality that matches our frequency into our lives. What you think about, what you become, and how you choose to live your life are dictated by your thoughts.

You'll attract another thought if you pay attention to one thought. You don't want to train your brain and make it more efficient at generating pessimistic and anxious thoughts.

Your brain is built to become more efficient at whatever you do over and over again. Choose your thoughts wisely, as positive thoughts are the key to positive change.

Whenever you wake up in the morning thinking it will be a bad day, it turns out to be your worst day ever. It's important to remember that energy attracts energy.

When this happens to you, try to change your thoughts by focusing on the good things in your life, writing them down, and being grateful.

Your vibration will shift to a higher frequency when you shift to a higher frequency, enabling you to attract positive, motivating people into your life, and opportunities will arise naturally.

Chapter 11: Conclusion

"One's dignity may be assaulted, vandalized, and cruelly mocked, but it cannot be taken away unless it is surrendered."

-Michael J. Fox

Every once in a while, we all need to be re-inspired and re-motivated.

And there are two ways to do that.

Firstly, talk to other people.

Others can motivate you. You know from experience that a great partner, a supportive family, or an encouraging boss can motivate you.

It's not a sad fact that "other" people want to motivate you, but to some extent, motivation has to come from within. You have to do things to motivate yourself and keep yourself motivated.

Motivation isn't magic, and it's not something that can be bought. Rather, you have to create it yourself, and everything that happens in your life is your doing.

You are essentially whom you make yourself to be, so everything is yours. You can only succeed if you can bounce back from failure, and that's motivation.

We all have those days when we're just not relaxed. Despite being mentally and physically exhausted, we get up and tackle the day.

And even when mentally upset, we don't have the luxury of staying in bed all day. Work and life are both parts of what we do. It's time to motivate ourselves and overcome the emotional hurdles when this happens.

Remember that most of the important things in the world were accomplished by people who didn't give up even when there was no hope.

It's not where a man stands in times of comfort and convenience but where he stands when things get tough and controversial. That's what really matters.

Embrace yourself even when nobody else does. You have to keep yourself motivated and happy. You don't have to rely on other people to keep you driven and happy. And yeah, movies, music, and meditation might help.

I think one can only be motivated once they are comfortable with who one is.

When you're comfortable in your skin, you don't have to be complacent with yourself. It doesn't mean you never need to change or never have to improve your life.

It doesn't mean you're narcissistic, arrogant, or prideful. As confidence plays a crucial role in self-love, it means you believe in yourself because you're more confident in yourself.

When you feel better about yourself, you tend to look and act better. Your actions, your demeanor, and your interactions with others will reflect how confident you are.

If you don't have confidence, you won't be able to recognize your worth and thrive. When you feel confident, you won't hesitate to stand up for yourself or try new things.

A person's attitude towards themselves and how others treat them will be directly related to how they feel about themselves.

If you don't feel confident, you're more likely to feel shy or unworthy of getting good things in your life.

Don't be afraid to stand out and be different- after all, these are the things that make you who you are. Get comfortable in your own skin.

Learn to love yourself unconditionally and practice self-care every day. You'll feel better in your own skin if you're comfortable with your body, your weaknesses, your failures, and so on.

Do you tend to compliment or critique your appearance when you look in the mirror? Do you talk about your fears or encourage yourself? When you look in the mirror, what do you think? Do you talk to yourself positively or negatively? Are you comfortable with your flaws? Do you talk life to yourself, or down talk yourself?

Body confidence isn't just about feeling good about yourself but about how you're doing in life as well. Feeling accomplished?

Are you moving forward and reaching your goals? Don't compare yourself to others because it'll leave you feeling empty inside.

Travel at your own pace and not others' pace. It's okay that some things take time, but you should keep working.

You may need to do some soul-searching to figure out why you feel inferior or lack self-confidence. You may be feeling low because of a past relationship, a trauma in your childhood, or voids in your life.

When you're true to yourself, you can build confidence. Look at each area of your life and figure out what to do next.

"To be beautiful means to be yourself. You don't need to be accepted by others. You need to accept yourself."

~Thich Nhat Hanh

One of the greatest factors of being comfortable in your own skin is being the kind of person you want to be. Having independence of thought, feeling, and action is a big part of being your own person.

That means you don't have to depend on others to tell you what to do, what to think, and what to do. Nevertheless, as John Donne famously said, "*No man is an island*," and "*happiness can't be found in isolation.*"

There's nothing wrong with being independent; you just don't have to live outside the boundaries of culture, society, and law; you don't have a character molded by socialization, or you're a bad person if you conform to everything.

People have a sphere of independent thinking and acting that can't be taken away from them without taking away their happiness.

It's true that people can feel so dependent on others that they don't know how to handle their lives. They feel lost, confused, manipulated, degraded, and needy.

It's possible for them to feel like something important is missing, but they don't know what's missing—let alone how to get it back.

Intimacy is one of the most common ways that people are manipulated by others, even if they know better.

It's hard for some people to plot an independent life plan because they'd rather live through someone else's accomplishments.

You should admire, be proud of, or be happy for someone else when they're doing well—more so than to envy, be jealous, or disdain them. You can't live through others without living through yourself, though. Happiness is generally promoted and sustained by the latter, not the former.

The classic song by Simon and Garfunkel says,

Hiding in my room,

safe within my womb,

I touch no one, and no one touches me.

I am a rock,

I'm an island.

A rock doesn't feel pain;

and an island doesn't cry

But that's more like a depressive thought than a healthy coping strategy.

Some people do the opposite of what they're supposed to for the sake of being oppositional, but that's not the case for everyone.

Besides being counterproductive, it's not based on logical decisions about what's in one's best interest.

Whenever you rely too much on others or conformity, you lose your sense of direction or purpose, but when you don't, you don't get anywhere.

As a matter of fact, there's a "*golden mean*" between relying on too much and too little. Nobody can achieve the perfect balance between these opposite poles, but being your own person requires getting a lot right.

You have to be interdependent with others if you want to live a balanced life. In accordance with your own freedom and others' freedom to forge respective life plans and make reasonable strides toward those plans, there's reciprocity between the support you receive from others and the support you give them.

The balance between helping others and living contentedly is obvious to you. You know when you have to draw the line between helping others and becoming a slave to them.

A relationship between independent individuals is intimate if each party serves their own interests and does not rely on the other for their own gratification.

Sexual intimacy is mutual gratification, and neither party serves the other. And to be able to reach the place where you can maintain that balance, you will need motivation.

Motivating ourselves can often be unpredictable, like the English sunshine; it can go from non-existent to appearing out of the blue.

Motivation is hard, but how can we keep our motivational drive strong to make sure it's there when we need it most, rather than relying on random bursts of motivation?

In order to live a successful life, you need to stay motivated for a long time. In spite of the failures and disappointments we're thrown into in life, self-motivation gives us the strength to keep moving forward.

Many people try to force themselves to get motivated by stuff they don't really care about. We need to do things for the right reasons.

Have a dream in sight or a rewarding goal in sight. Nobody really wants to get up early. When you wake up early, you'll suddenly be motivated and focused.

The biggest motivation killer of all is a lack of self-belief. If you don't believe in yourself, you won't fail or be disappointed.

It's more common for people to focus on their weaknesses and obstacles rather than their strengths and abilities. They're the ones who are responsible for their lack of success.

If you want to get yourself out of your slump, remind yourself how far you have already come. Instead of dwelling on how far you still have to go, remember just how far you have already come.

You should begin to feel amazed by how competent and successful you have already proven yourself to be if you do this.

When it comes to deceiving ourselves and making up stories that are not based on facts, we are often our own worst enemies. A negative interpretation of a situation will lead us to search for evidence in our reality to support that narrative.

Motivate yourself and boost your confidence by telling yourself an entirely different story, one that is more optimistic.

Write down your strengths, your achievements, and your advantages. This should motivate you and give you the kick-start you need to achieve your goals.

Motivate yourself with the end goal in mind, not with the fear of failure. The key now is to develop a direction to help guide you toward your goals as you gain focus on what you want, whether you are aiming to lose weight or have eyes for your desired position in your career.

When you want to reach your personal goals, set small, measurable goals that you can hit every day. Overwhelming and burnout are the enemies of self-motivation. So, avoid scaring yourself before you get started.

There will be times when we all feel tired and low on energy. It is important to accept that these times are to be expected and to take them in stride.

When we are experiencing these occasional slumps, it is important to silence our negative thoughts and nurture our motivating ones so that we can gain momentum when we need it most.

We need to manifest what we desire. It helps us overcome our negative energy and heighten our spirituality.

We attract more of what we put out when we create thoughts of lack and emptiness. When we move to thoughts of giving and sharing, we receive the same energy back.

You have the power to manifest what you think. Your every action, behavior, and choice is dictated by your thoughts, so when you align your thoughts and emotions with positive vibrations and states of being, you are better equipped to make choices that result in the manifestation of what you want.

There's no doubt that the concept of manifestation and the law of attraction is enticing. After all, simply thinking something into existence seems like a pretty good deal. But unfortunately, it's never that simple.

It is true that changing your mindset can be a powerful tool for attracting the things you desire, but it is also not a substitute for taking the necessary actions in order to achieve them.

If despite your best efforts, you cannot manifest what you want through the law of attraction, you should not blame yourself and your misguided thinking.

People would be manifesting with great success if it were that simple, but that is not the case. And manifesting can be challenging for a variety of reasons.

One thing to keep in mind is that the universe is unlikely to grant your request if it isn't for everybody's highest good.

Additionally, you will find it much harder to make your request come true if you are not specific about what you're asking for or don't really know how it will feel or look like.

You must also believe yourself capable of achieving what you ask for. If your conscious and unconscious minds agree, that's a problem that can prevent you from manifesting your desires.

I think people believe that manifesting will show up exactly the way they imagine it, but that's not always true. The universe often gives us something, but we don't let it because we're too fixated on how it should show up. Manifestation requires being open to unanticipated synchronicities and possibilities.

Get clear on how you want your goal or desire to look and feel, and you'll be able to tap into the power of manifestation.

It's similar to vision boards, where you create a physical representation of your goals, and visualization works the same way, although it's internal rather than external.

You can do either to get a better sense of what you're asking for and align yourself more with what you're doing. It's often hardest for people to believe that they can manifest.

In order to experiment with the law of attraction, you need to, for a short time, eradicate your doubts and believe in your mind and feel (in your heart and body) that you have what you're asking for already.

You can start by making believe if you don't believe it. Act as if you have it now, and as you do, you'll start believing.

Think about what you want, and you will attract what you want into your life. Since thoughts are powerful, you're changing your thoughts to bring exactly what you want into your life.

Start feeling what your success will feel like once it arrives. Feel and believe it with your heart, mind, body, and soul.

Try to imagine what you're going to feel like when you get what you asked for: What's it going to look like? How will it feel? How does it sound? How will it smell? How will it taste?

Imagine yourself getting what you want with the mantra: *"I'm getting this now. I'm getting that now."* Feel it as though you've already gotten it.

Your life will be more positive when you focus on the abundance in your life. If you only think about what's wrong in life and focus on what's lacking, you're gonna attract negativity to your life, and you'll keep chasing what you want most.

People who complain a lot usually attract friends and followers who complain too. People who are happy and energetic will attract people who are also motivated and driven.

This is what the Universal Law of Attraction looks like in action!

I want to emphasize that the Universe doesn't care what kind of vibration you send out. It doesn't really matter whether you are positive or negative. It just responds to what you offer.

By changing your vibration, you can change how the universe responds to you! By creating vibrations that reflect your desires, you can manifest specific outcomes in your life!

The key to doing this is living in constant awareness of your energy, thoughts, and feelings - and how they form your reality in seven different ways.

A growth mindset has mental health benefits, too. It can reduce stress, prevent depression, and help to manage stress. A positive attitude can promote better physical health, longer life, and even lower cholesterol levels.

As a result of this improved emotional state, you'll be able to develop more skills, which will lead to greater success. Ultimately, you'll be more mindful, grateful, and compassionate towards yourself as well.

Basically, the law of attraction states that whatever you focus your energy on will get back to you in the form of positive energy. By focusing on what you want to achieve, you'll emit positive energy that attracts those achievements.

A positive attitude and an optimistic mindset can be credited with the law of attraction, which advocates of self-help and self-care consider natural law.

In the same vein, a positive attitude is not synonymous with relentless, toxic positivity. There's space for acknowledging reality, and reality doesn't always go our way every day.

Setbacks occur. It is possible to rise above setbacks if we are optimistic. If you are optimistic, you don't have to believe that "everything will work out" if you believe enough.

The optimistic mindset is a mindset based on the belief that there is a solution or a way to overcome a challenge. This mindset combines hope and action for problem-solving.

Dreams don't work much unless you do them. Positive thinking is one thing, but it doesn't get you anywhere. That's not what the law of attraction is about.

It's all about action, planning, and positive thinking. Your positive attitude will definitely benefit you in the future. And you'll see what you've attracted from your positive attitude and action-filled behaviors one day.

If you've heard the Law of Attraction, you might have also heard that visualization is a big deal.

Law of Attraction Visualization success depends on using it correctly. What you don't hear is that you have to visualize your desire in order to attract your desire.

Visualization techniques for the Law of Attraction aren't like ordinary meditation or basic visualization techniques. They're more than just using your mind to imagine yourself succeeding.

It's not like watching yourself on TV. The energy doesn't come from your mind.

In the Law of Attraction visualization, your heart is at the center of it all...and you can use it to manifest what you desire.

If a person visualizes the Law of Attraction correctly, it feels like falling in love. With your eyes, ears, and mouth on the scene, you see, hear, and taste everything.

There's no outside vantage point. You are experiencing the experience as if it were as real as you, as real as the screen or page where you arc reading these words... It's as if your visualization is the only thing that exists.

When you lie in bed, you have the best chance of experiencing the Law of Attraction visualization properly.

Close your eyes and let your mind wander. Imagine lying in bed in your new house. Smell the detergent that was used to wash your sheets. Feel the sheets on your skin and the pillow under your head. Feel the gentle breeze coming through your windows and drifting over your skin. Hear your partner breathing softly next to you...

Think about sitting in front of a fire with a hot cup of hot chocolate in your hands. Take a cup and hold it up to your nose and breathe in the delicious smell of chocolate. Hear the crackling of the fire as it is held up. Feel the heat of the fire as it comes off. Look over at your family planning your skiing trip tomorrow. Listen to them laugh. Feel the chocolate hit your lips, drift seductively across your tongue, and flow warmly down your throat as you drink it.

Allow yourself to be immersed in the scene.

Using your visualization of the Law of Attraction, think about what you want to achieve.

Consider the possibility of how you might use it. Consider the possibilities of what it might enable you to do. Go beyond just having something.

Embrace the vision, give it a lot of love, and take it as far as you can. Enjoy it, and be true to what you want to accomplish.

Keep your eyes on it. Let the Universe take care of the rest. You will find that your dream will come true.

Everyone possesses the creative ability of visualization. Its general use is to explore possibilities and experiment with interacting with them.

The method is also useful for practicing new or improved behaviors, such as improving athletic ability or preparing for a speech.

You can visualize intelligently or unintelligently, like many abilities. When you use your imagination to think about your worst fears or disasters, you elaborate and intensify your problems.

It's a bad idea to use your imagination in this way. Rationalizing that you're just preparing for the worst is, at best, a very weak argument.

Luckily, we can use constructive imagination to explore our future in more helpful ways. Let's say we were more calm, cheerful and confident.

If we performed an imaginary rehearsal of what it would be like to move through our day with more self-control and optimism, we could visualize this state in more detail. In creating a visualization, we're bridging the present with the future, bringing familiarity and the unknown together.

Using our imagination, we can project our energy into thought forms to represent the things we're going to see and do.

Our minds invest mental power into these thought forms when we use them to imagine a positive outcome. They then act as "batteries" for changing attitudes and behavior.

It's not always necessary to visualize in meditation, but it makes exploring mental vistas a little less weird. In order to explore new possibilities, we need to create an image.

First, it stabilizes our focus of interest as a place we associate with healing, peace, or education. Second, we anchor this place mentally in a meditative state, so we can come back whenever we want.

They see a clear image in their minds of what they're focusing on. There's nothing wrong with intellectuals thinking about things and the ideas they entertain. They do visualize, but it's a mistake to think they don't. Symbolizing what they're thinking about with an image is like recalling a memory or symbol for it.

The people who're not concrete visualizers often claim they don't visualize at all. It's similar to recalling a memory of what they saw, but they can explain the dashboard of their car or the colors in their bathroom. Imagining speculating about their options or exploring new possibilities is also how they visualize.

In other words, if the mental imager is asked to imagine a rose or blond Labrador dog, it's easy for them to do. If they're asked to visualize a Dalmatian with red spots instead of black spots, they can do it.

A pink elephant outside your door is one of the best ways for these types to master visualization, so they avoid it at all costs.

The use of our mind intelligently is linked to our higher potential in meditative states by visualizing them. It's easy to build a figurative bridge between what we know and what we don't.

By doing so, we're able to connect the abstract with our concrete thinking. By remembering or seeing a phone or computer, we can get new insights and information.

We can absorb a peaceful mood by imagining a tranquil landscape. Our mental symbols can be a doorway to new emotions, ideas, and abstract concepts.

Having a visual aid also helps us stay focused and stable so we can keep up with abstract and new forces. It creates a place within us where we can come and experience new things.

Finally, one thing I would like to share with you is that when things go wrong in your day, it's hard to shift your mind, so just take a nap or go to sleep and then smile at the universe the next day because you're a living thing and start the day with new positive energy.

Self-love is the key to strength, and courage is the key to being your own person. Rather than being influenced by outside events, you are in control of your mind.

Realize this, and you'll be able to handle anything. Life is not unbearable because of circumstances; it is unbearable because you lack meaning and purpose. Knowing is freedom, so learning is the highest thing you can do.

We are not human beings having a spiritual experience. We are spiritual beings having a human experience. Don't waste what you've got by wanting what you don't have. You've already received so much, but that doesn't mean you're done.

I can. Therefore, I am.

-Simone Weil

www.ingramcontent.com/pod-product-compliance
Lightning Source LLC
Chambersburg PA
CBHW061600250726
48657CB00020B/214